"Dr. Baumann literally 'wrote the book' on cosmetic dermatology; her manual is the first on the shelf for every practicing dermatologist. I'm excited that she has now made her unique understanding of what the skin needs to look younger and healthier available for the public. The Baumann system is an easy-to-use program that is beneficial for people of all colors and skin types."

—SUSAN C. TAYLOR, M.D., founding director, Skin of Color Center of St. Luke's Roosevelt Hospital Center, and author of *Brown Skin*

"*The Skin Type Solution* is the best book I've read on skin care. Every recommendation reflects current state-of-the-art information and research. Baumann's skin-typing profiles are so well organized with precise detail that virtually any reader will be able to identify her type of skin and then choose products that really work."

—PAULA BEGOUN, author of
*Don't Go to the Cosmetics Counter Without Me*

"Consumers today are bombarded with information that raises endless questions: Should you use soap? Does eye cream really work? What is the best moisturizer? If your world is crowded with too many confusing beauty regimens and skin care choices, Dr. Baumann provides a highly reliable road map to healthy skin."

—DAVID J. LEFFELL, M.D., professor of dermatology and surgery, Yale School of Medicine, and author of *Total Skin*

# THE
# SKIN TYPE
# SOLUTION

# THE
# SKIN TYPE
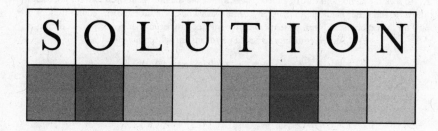

## LESLIE BAUMANN, M.D.

BANTAM BOOKS
TRADE PAPERBACKS
NEW YORK

The material in this book is for informational purposes, and is not intended to replace the services of a licensed dermatologist or other appropriate health care professional. Readers are encouraged to seek the advice and care of a medical doctor for the diagnosis and treatment of illnesses, diseases, and other medical problems and conditions. The case studies portrayed in this book are based on the experiences of real patients, whose identities have been changed to protect their privacy. Any resemblance to actual persons is entirely coincidental.

2010 Bantam Books Trade Paperback Edition

Copyright © 2006, 2007, and 2010 by MetaBeauty, Inc.

Published in the United States by Bantam Books, an imprint of
The Random House Publishing Group, a division of Random House, Inc., New York.

BANTAM BOOKS and the rooster colophon are registered trademarks of Random House, Inc.

Originally published in hardcover in the United States by Bantam Books, an imprint of
The Random House Publishing Group, a division of Random House, Inc., in 2006.

ISBN 978-0-553-38330-0

Printed in the United States of America

www.bantamdell.com

2 4 6 8 9 7 5 3 1

*This book is dedicated to my wonderful family:*
*Roger, Robert, and Max Baumann,*
*and anyone who has ever suffered an embarrassing bad skin day.*

# CONTENTS

# ACKNOWLEDGMENTS

Many people contributed directly or indirectly to this book and I am extremely grateful for everyone's help. First, I want to thank my patients, friends, family, and colleagues who patiently answered questionnaire after questionnaire over the years until I got it right. The original version contained over two hundred questions, requiring quite a commitment on their part. I offer tremendous thanks to the questionnaire experts who gave me excellent advice about questionnaire development, including Dr. David Lee and Dr. Frangchao Ma in the Department of Epidemiology at the University of Miami. Special thanks to Sharon Jacob, M.D., an expert on contact dermatitis at the University of Miami who helped me develop the questions covering skin allergies and sensitivity.

Thanks to all of the companies that sent skin care products to be studied and evaluated. I also thank my patients, family, and friends who used these skin care products and reported back to me about their experiences. Some of them suffered redness, acne, rashes, and itching in the name of Skin Type science. What troupers!

Thanks to Nikki at Brownes & Co. in Miami Beach for letting me spend hours looking at skin care products and for letting me use her beautiful store as a background in my picture in this book.

Thanks to my staff for putting up with me during the years leading up to the publication of this book. Thanks for being flexible, hardworking, and dependable. Susan Schaffer and Laura Black suffered the most and I can't thank them enough. Susan, you're a great friend and colleague. Tere Calcines was always there for me when I needed help. I'm also grateful to Denese, Marie, Franshely, Vanessa, Conchita, Clara, Debra, Olga, Jussane, Jasmine, and all the others who worked or volunteered in my office. My fellows—Esperanza Welsh, Lucy Martin, Monica Halem, Justin Vujevich, Anele Slezinger, and Melissa Lazarus—were terrific.

Special thanks to Joy Bryde, who organized my life and whose teachings helped shape the development of this book.

Many people mentored me in my career, but each of the following people selflessly taught me and guided me to this point: Ben Smith, M.D.; Francisco Kerdel, M.D.; William Eaglstein, M.D.; Larry Schachner, M.D.; Steve Mandy, M.D.; Jim Leyden, M.D.; Joseph Jorizzo, M.D.; and David Leffell, M.D.

Thanks to Richard Pine and Catherine Drayton, my incredible agents at Inkwell Management, and Alison Rose Levy, a great friend and a true pleasure to work with—you all are the best. This book would not have happened without you. To my new friends at Bantam Dell—including Irwyn Applebaum, Nita Taublib, Betsy Hulsebosch, Cynthia Lasky, Carolyn Schwartz, and Philip Rappaport—I offer thanks for the opportunity and your enthusiasm. I hope that we have many more chances to work together. Thanks to Bantam's publicity team—Barb Burg and Theresa Zoro—and to Sandi Mendelson for performing PR magic.

And last, but certainly not least, I want to thank my loving family. My parents, Lynn and Jack McClendon, and in-laws, Josie and David Kenin, helped me on every level possible. My husband, Roger, who has been by my side for the last sixteen years; and my two sons, Robert and Max, who bring happiness, fun, and tons of love to my life. I adore you all and wish you all a lifetime of great skin!

## AUTHOR'S NOTE

I would like to thank all of the visitors to www.skintypesolutions.com, who provided suggestions and favorite product names for this paperback edition. The book has been streamlined to make it easier to carry with you to the store and many new products and Baumann choices have been added. I would like to express endless gratitude to my aesthetician Robyn Vandenberg who taught the Baumann Skin Typing System to her students before joining me in 2008. She has been a huge asset in helping me identify exciting new products and type them for the correct skin type. She also keeps our followers up to date at www.Facebook.com/BaumannCosmetic. Thanks to Robyn and our Facebook friends and website visitors for helping me choose the products in this new edition.

Thank you for being a part of this Skin Type Revolution!

Affectionately,

Leslie Baumann, M.D.

## PART ONE

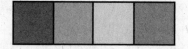

# The Skin Type
# Revolution

CHAPTER ONE

# Why Skin Typing?

◼

## INTRODUCTION

How many times have you gone to a cosmetic counter and spent $50 to $150 on products you never again use? Has a saleswoman or cosmetologist sold you a line that "did wonders for me," but does nothing for you? Have you developed an allergy or irritation to a product without knowing the cause? Why does your best friend swear by a facial care product that makes your skin look and feel terrible? Should you or shouldn't you use soap? Why do you hate the feel of sunscreen, though you know you should use it? Is a chemical face peel right for you? Should you consider using Retin-A?

If you owned a Subaru Forester, you wouldn't follow the maintenance procedures for a Volkswagen Golf. So if you happen to have dry, sensitive skin, why on earth would you use a moisturizer, cleanser, and cosmetic procedure more suited to someone with oily, resistant skin?

The reason? You don't know what type of skin you have; therefore, you don't know how to care for your skin. Until the publication of *The Skin Type Solution,* the Baumann Skin Typing System was not widely known or available. While many people have a general understanding of their skin, most have relied on commonly known but imprecise, unscientific definitions that fall short of providing a true and complete picture.

My many years as a dermatologist, researcher, and professor of dermatology have convinced me that no one ever needs to have a "bad skin day." Knowing your Skin Type is the missing, essential step to finding your way to beneficial products and treatments—and beautiful skin. But if you're like the typical first-time patient at my bustling Baumann Cosmetic & Research Institute, I'll bet you:

- Don't know your Skin Type
- Don't know that it's essential to base skin care decisions on your Skin Type

- Use the wrong products for your Skin Type
- Spend much more than you should on those products
- Use the wrong procedures for your Skin Type
- Fail to take advantage of procedures that would benefit your Skin Type

When it comes to using skin care products and services, most people have been in the Dark Ages, wandering through a maze of product misinformation and overzealous marketing, lucky to stumble on anything that works.

To properly care for your skin and prevent aging, you need a treatment model that describes and captures the very real and scientifically verifiable distinctions in skin physiology.

Skin Typing does just that.

Plus, you need a concrete program specifically and individually tailored to the unique attributes of *your* Skin Type. *The Skin Type Solution* provides all of that vital information and guidance.

**Once you've discovered your Skin Type (through answering a questionnaire in Chapter Three), you can go straight to the chapter on your Skin Type and find everything you need right there.** There is a science to skin care, and once you know your Skin Type, it all gets a lot easier.

I've spent the last thirteen years defining and clinically testing my Skin Type solutions on tens of thousands of patients at my University of Miami clinic and the Baumann Cosmetic and Research Institute to assure that my scientific criteria will work for everyone, of every skin color, ethnicity, age, and sex. And it does.

Perhaps you've already benefited from understanding your psychological type, your learning style, or your Ayurvedic type. If so, you'll appreciate how critical it is to get a handle on your Skin Type. This understanding lets you take control of your skin.

## MY SPECIAL EXPERTISE

The guidance and gems I'll give you won't appear anywhere else. I launched, and for thirteen years directed, the University of Miami Cosmetic Center, the first university-run cosmetic research center in the United States, where I treated thousands of patients every year. In addition to being an M.D., I was a professor at the University of Miami and the chief of the Division of Cosmetic Dermatology, making me the first cosmetic dermatologist in the United States dedicated to the field of cosmetic dermatology who is also a full-time university faculty member, teaching and conducting research.

This unprecedented combination affords me a unique position. My academic responsibilities keep me right on the cutting edge of research, while my clinical work has been a proving ground for refining the recommendations that arise from my findings.

My clients—who range from gorgeous fashion models to topflight professionals, to fellow physicians, to all kinds of men and women concerned about aging—have reaped the benefits of my unique understanding of the role of Skin Type in skin care.

As a scientist who is also a woman who loves to experiment with beauty and skin care products and routines, I'm tireless in seeking out and researching all beauty options because I use them myself. What's more, as a person who wants to look my best all my life, I can put myself in your shoes and figure out how to best serve your skin care needs.

## Defining a New Typology

Up until now, the field of dermatology lacked a rational model that people could learn to follow and apply for themselves. Prior to Skin Typing, the preexisting mode of analyzing skin differences dated back to the early 1900s, when cosmetic giant Helena Rubenstein first divided skin into four categories: normal, combination, dry, and sensitive. While that was revolutionary for its time, today we can apply more accurate scientific criteria to the range of skin differences.

Before Skin Typing, even dermatologists felt frustrated, since we all want to understand skin better and offer our patients tailor-made solutions. But until now, the revolutionary classification of the sixteen Skin Types was not there to help.

Here's just one example of the kind of confusion that runs rampant, even among professionals. I recently was on the advisory board of a major company with two prominent dermatologists. One was an "R" (someone with resistant, nonreactive skin) and the other one was an "S" (someone with sensitive skin). Right there in front of the company president, the two had a huge argument, with the "R" dermatologist claiming that there was no difference in skin care products and that it was all marketing hype. She could use anything on her facial skin, she told us, even Ivory soap, without a problem. The "S" skin dermatologist was shocked. Almost everything made her skin turn red and sting, she retorted. These two skin professionals did not understand that their opposing points of view stemmed from their opposite Skin Types. I saw very clearly that something was missing and wanted to simplify skin care, once and for all.

As a clinician, I'd seen the damage caused by following an inappropriate skin care routine. As a caring doctor, I'd heard the frustration and confusion of people trying to make good skin care choices while barraged by a plethora of products and overwhelmed by conflicting and often misleading marketing claims. Because each person had particular skin care needs, I noticed that the same products did not work for everyone, so I tailored individualized skin care regimens for my clients. Over time a clear, consistent, and replicable typology emerged. The sixteen Skin Types are the keys to a complete diagnostic and treatment program that covers every significant skin factor and that *really works*.

My system measures four factors in skin: oiliness vs. dryness, resistance vs. sensitivity, pigmentation vs. non-pigmentation, and tightness vs. wrinkling. Determining where you fall in each of the four categories serves as the foundation for typing your skin. Your Skin Type is more than the sum of the four different factors. Their interplay and expression are unique for each type. After seeing literally thousands of patients and refining the Baumann Skin Type Questionnaire over the last ten years, I can assure you that Skin Typing captures each Skin Type's unique qualities and shows you how to work with your type's strengths and weaknesses.

Once you understand your Skin Type, proper skin care isn't complicated or costly. You won't need to use a shelfful of products. Honing in on what your skin needs will actually simplify your beauty routine, making it easier to follow and more economical. Following the advice I'll extend in your Skin Type's chapter will end "bad skin days" because it will end bad skin care decisions.

## HOW TO USE THIS BOOK

In reading the opening chapter of this book, you'll familiarize yourself with the underlying principles of Skin Typing. In Chapter Two, you'll learn my innovative vocabulary to help you understand the different factors that I take into account when determining your Skin Type. In Chapter Three, you'll take the Baumann Skin Type Questionnaire. Once you tabulate your results, you will know exactly which one of the sixteen types describes your skin. You can then turn directly to that chapter for a complete profile that will provide you with everything you need to take charge of your skin and give it the best possible care. The bottom line is that by reading your chapter, you will get to know your skin. This will provide the foundation for following my subsequent advice.

Each chapter contains Daily Skin Care Regimens specifically designed to address your Skin Type's problem areas. To follow your type's regimen, you will need to use the kinds of products I recommend. I'll provide a list of suggestions for each type of product, as well as extra suggestions to use when you have specific skin problems.

If you currently use products that you find effective, you can also continue to use them, if you wish. However, if you decide to do that, I advise you to consult the lists of ingredients that define which ones are favorable or counterproductive for your Skin Type. Some ingredients may be helpful for one of your skin concerns, but exacerbate another skin problem. For example, genistein, a component found in soy, helps wrinkles, but also increases pigmentation. A Non-Pigmented, Wrinkled Skin Type could safely use it, but a Pigmented, Wrinkled Type should use only products that contain soy that has had the genistein removed. That's one reason why I advise that you double-check your current products to ensure that they do not contain any no-nos. If they do, I recommend that you change products, as you could be unwittingly causing a problem. And you may also find that some of your favorite products do indeed contain helpful ingredients for your type. Still, I can best guarantee results with the products I know and recommend.

This book should be your companion when you shop for skin care products. As you put my recommendations in place, monitor how well they are working for you to assess whether or not consulting a dermatologist would be of benefit. For some Skin Types, I provide one or more additional Stage Two Daily Skin Care Regimens that address treating special skin problems. Near the end of each chapter, I will point you toward your best options in cosmetic dermatology.

In the chapter on your Skin Type, you will find:

1. Understanding of:
    a. The basic qualities of your Skin Type
    b. Your Skin Type's issues and challenges
    c. Risk factors associated with your Skin Type

2. Guidelines for:
    a. Your Skin Type's Daily Skin Care Regimen
    b. Sun protection for your skin
    c. Makeup that will help improve your skin condition
    d. Cosmetic procedures that can help your skin (where applicable)
    e. Cosmetic procedures that are not recommended for you (where applicable)

3. Specific Recommendations for:
   a. Skin care products for your daily skin care routine
   b. Skin care ingredients (to look for on product labels) that address your key
      skin issues
   c. Skin care ingredients (to look for on product labels) that you should
      avoid because they can worsen your skin

My role in research and industry development gives me an unparalleled across-the-board knowledge of skin care ingredients.

I'll indicate the best way to cleanse your skin, reveal whether you need to use a toner or a moisturizer, diagnose whether exfoliation is advisable for you, and advise you when you'd benefit from prescription skin medications. All of my product recommendations will include options at low, medium, and high prices so that whatever your budget, you can follow my recommendations to successful skin care. All selections are widely available, so you'll have no trouble obtaining them.

Your Skin Type chapter will also help you to avoid products and procedures that—while recommended for other types—are either useless or potentially harmful for you. If you are curious about a cosmetic procedure, like Botox, your chapter will indicate whether, based on your Skin Type, it's something that you and your dermatologist should consider. That way you can make sure you choose the skin procedures most beneficial for your skin's particular needs.

## WHEN TO CONSULT A DERMATOLOGIST

In addition to guiding you through the product maze, I will help you decide when to consult a dermatologist. Some types have very little need to see a doctor, while certain others really benefit from the prescription medications, light treatments, and other procedures doctors can provide. In fact, for certain Skin Types with increased skin issues, nonprescription products may not be sufficiently effective. People with highly resistant skin, for example, need higher-octane products, which only licensed physicians can prescribe.

Due to a national shortage of qualified dermatologists, people wait an average of three months to get an appointment. As a result, most dermatologists cannot always spend the time necessary to address basic skin care needs. By teaching you how to meet your basic skin care needs without a dermatologist, I'll ensure you make efficient use of your valuable appointment time when you see a doctor.

Finally, I have launched a website, www.skintypesolutions.com, to track your responses to different products, so now you can join the patients who see me at my clinic in offering your feedback and experiences while following the Baumann Skin Type Solution. Log on to www.skintypesolutions .com and share your skin care discoveries with me and other people from around the world who share your Skin Type. Find out what's new and ask specific questions about your skin concerns. You can also watch for our PBS special that will air in December 2010 called *The Skin Type Solution.*

## What You Need to Know About Skin Care Products

For you as a consumer in the billion-dollar skin care industry, lack of information about products is costly, and you have to bridge the gap between what you *know* and what you *need to know.* Without accurate information, you are throwing your money away, because you are completely at the mercy of advertisers and marketers. With the specific information about your skin's needs explained in this book, you can take control of your skin.

This book will save you the expense, trouble, and waste of buying the wrong products—while directing you to the right ones. My recommendations are ingredient driven, and once you've learned my criteria, you too will be better able to read a cosmetic label and figure out if it's appropriate for you.

I have tried to incorporate into this book every kind of skin care product that I feel is useful, limiting the scope to facial care products. I have chosen the products recommended in this book based on their ingredients, manufacturing practices, and formulations.

Instead of letting you waste your valuable time and money tracking down products that wind up in the trash, I will direct you to ones that will really help. I've reviewed the clinical trial data for the products, when available, to offer those proven effective. Finally, since my patients have used my recommendations, I've listened to their feedback and tracked their treatment results to guarantee the efficacy of the treatment approach and product selection for each Skin Type. All you have to do is take the test, determine your Skin Type, and choose from the products in your chapter. And at least when you splurge on products and procedures, you'll know you are getting your money's worth.

The recommendations are independent of any relationships that I have with the companies that manufacture them. Of course, when I work with a company, I know more about its products. However, I work with over forty-two companies and have approached many others for information while writing this book. In addition, when I find products with helpful ingredients from other sources, like stores or the Internet, I test them as well. After all, I test skin care products for a living—so why not?

All the products that I recommend:

1. Contain the right ingredients for your Skin Type
2. Contain sufficient amounts of active ingredients to be effective
3. Do not contain counterproductive ingredients
4. Are formulated effectively for your needs
5. Are packaged to maintain stability of the active ingredients
6. Are cosmetically elegant (smell good and feel good)
7. Got a thumbs-up from those who've used them
8. Are easily available for purchase

Finally, since all products meet all of the above criteria, I often pick the cheapest option (or a hands-down favorite) as a Baumann's Choice. This designates the best value to make your product selections easier.

## SKIN TYPING IS UNIVERSAL

One of the fascinating features of Skin Typing is that people of different ethnic or racial backgrounds can share a Skin Type. In most instances, all people with the same Skin Type will follow the exact same treatment plan, but sometimes skin color can be a differentiating factor because of the way pigment (the factor in skin that produces color) is produced in different racial and ethnic groups. For example, two best friends, Valerie, a medium–skin-toned brunette, and Dana, a dark-skinned woman, came in for back-to-back appointments. After they each took the questionnaire and tabulated their results, they were surprised to discover that they shared the same Skin Type. They were both "P," Pigmented Skin Types, which gave both Valerie and Dana a tendency to develop pigmentation issues. And each of them *did* have a problem with pigmentation. That's why they came to my office.

Valerie had an area of dark skin discoloration (called melasma) on her cheek, and Dana had dark spots in areas where she had once had pimples. Although I recommended that they follow the exact same protocol and use the same kinds of products, there was one key difference. Valerie could benefit from an advanced cosmetic procedure that uses light instruments or lasers to treat pigment problems like hers, while Dana would benefit most from prescription products used daily and should not undergo laser treatment since this can cause discoloration in people with darker skin tones.

That's why, throughout the book whenever an adjustment based on skin color is needed, I'll fine-tune recommendations so that you will know how to adapt them to your needs whether you have a light, medium, or dark skin tone.

## SKIN CARE MYTHS

When people come into my office, I regularly have to deprogram them of skin care *dis*-information. For example, do you buy into any of these common beauty myths?

Myth #1: *The way to find the right skin care product is by buying lots of different products until you find one that works for you (if you're lucky).*

Actually, this approach works well for the cosmetics industry, but it's not so good for you—unless you happen to have loads of money, tons of free time, and a desire to experiment on your skin. Yet, that's the way most people purchase skin care products and services. Without knowing your Skin Type and being directed to the range of products that work well for it, you are at the mercy of marketers and advertisers.

In this book, I will demystify skin products, and let you know what's worthwhile, or worthless, for your Skin Type's needs—and why. Because of the way that they are regulated by the FDA, cosmetic companies cannot lay claim to any biological activity. If they did, their products would be regulated as drugs, with costly clinical trials needed to validate their claims. Instead they make vague marketing statements. No wonder people are confused. However, as a dermatologist, I can reveal the biological effects of different products to cut through the hype.

Myth #2: *The more expensive a product, the better it will work.*

What does the high price tag on that designer skin cream buy you? It is not always the ingredients in the bottle. In some cases you are footing the bill for the marketing and bottling of that product. In fact, if tomorrow someone invented the world's best skin cream, how would you know if it is worth the cost? Knowing your skin type and visiting www.skintypesolutions.com will help you stay current so you will know what products really work for your specific Baumann Skin Type. Some day I'd love to see high-end lines that are really worth the extra expense because they are packed with ingredients that can deliver real results. In this book, you'll learn what products are worth splurging for and when you can choose a cheaper option.

Myth #3: *Ivory soap is for sensitive skin.*

Any product that vigorously suds and foams contains detergent, a strict no-no for dry skin. The best-known example is Ivory soap, marketed with the buzz phrase "so pure it floats." Advertising featured pictures of delicate babies and fair-skinned blondes, along with the recommendation that since it was "pure, and fragrance free," it was designed "for sensitive skin." Nothing could be further from the truth. Vigorously foaming soaps, like Ivory, are terrible for dry skin because they wash away the natural lipids that help your skin retain moisture. If you have dry skin, never use anything that makes a lot of bubbles, especially bubble bath. Thin foam and thin bubbles are all right. *Never* wash your face with shampoo no matter what your Skin Type. Instead use non-foaming cleansers or minimally foaming cleansers like Cetaphil, Dove, Pond's, or certain Nivea products.

Myth #4: *The food I eat won't affect my skin.*

Your diet does impact your skin, and there's no doubt that going on a no- or low-fat diet can increase skin dryness. Studies have shown that patients on cholesterol-lowering drugs often suffer from dry skin. Cholesterol is actually an important part of the skin that helps it remain hydrated.

Myth #5: *Paying attention to my skin is a waste of time.*

If you have one of the easier Skin Types, your recommended routine is not going to create unnecessary complexity. What's more, fine-tuning your skin care can only save you money and optimize your skin in the long run. On the other hand, if you have a challenging Skin Type, treating your skin right and preventing future problems is an absolute essential. Most skin problems are better addressed sooner rather than later. And whatever your age, skin condition, or Skin Type, sooner is today.

## READY, SET . . . SKIN TYPE!

I'm truly delighted to be able to share with you my discoveries and to help you manage your skin and treat it right. Try the regimens and products, and see how they work for you. Don't hesitate to see a dermatologist if you need to, as there are many advanced medications and procedures of real benefit. Finally, share Skin Typing with your friends, family, and loved ones because there's a Skin Type Solution for everyone.

# CHAPTER TWO

# Understanding Skin Type Categories

■

In Chapter Three, you will take the Baumann Skin Type Questionnaire to identify the four dominant factors that determine your Skin Type. These factors are: oily vs. dry, sensitive vs. resistant, pigmented vs. non-pigmented, and wrinkled vs. tight. But first, in this chapter, I'll offer some basic wisdom about each of these factors, as well as provide the science behind them. The key factors interact to determine the skin's appearance, problems, needs, and vulnerabilities, and therefore dictate the kinds of products, ingredients, and treatments useful to address them. To get started, let me introduce you to some basics about the skin.

## THE BIOLOGY OF THE SKIN

The top layer of the skin, called the epidermis, is made up of four distinct layers. When you look at someone's skin, you see the very top layer, made up of cells that reflect light. When that top layer is smooth, it reflects light evenly so that the skin looks more uniform and radiant than it does when the surface is rougher.

At the lowest portion of the epidermis are "mother cells," called basal cells, which produce all the other skin cells. They divide into "daughter cells," which rise up to the higher levels of the epidermis. As they travel, they age and eventually die, so that the top layer consists of dead cells that naturally exfoliate off in a process called the "cell cycle," which can take anywhere from twenty-six to forty-two days. Between the third and eighth decades of life, the cell cycle slows from 30 to 50 percent of its pace in youth. That means that older skin renews itself much more slowly, forming a rough surface of cells, rather than a smooth surface.

The uppermost cells contain a natural moisturizing factor (NMF), which holds moisture. The body responds to a dry environment by producing more NMF, but it takes several days for production to rev up, so your skin may become quite dehydrated before help comes. That's why it's important to moisturize your skin in any dry environment.

Substances released by the cells in the middle of the epidermis form a protective film made of lipids (fats) that surrounds skin cells and helps keep the skin hydrated. Your fingers and toes contain fewer lipids and are therefore not as "watertight" as your legs, which is why your fingers and toes look shriveled after immersion in water but your legs do not. Your skin cracks in cold weather because the chilled lipids become stiffer and less able to adjust to movement. The goal of the best moisturizers is to increase the amount of these important lipids, helping your skin to hold moisture.

## FACTOR ONE: SKIN HYDRATION: OILY VS. DRY

With oily skin, your face may often look shiny, and you naturally avoid products that feel oily. You'll be more vulnerable to acne and breakouts than Dry Skin Types. People with dry skin will notice that their skin feels dry, and has a dull color and/or rough texture.

Dryness and oiliness depend primarily on the condition of the skin barrier, the outer layer of skin that helps the skin retain moisture, and the oil (sebum) production itself.

The barrier is like a brick wall, with each brick (or cell) held in place by mortar (fats called lipids). Harmful ingredients, cold and dry weather can wear down these fats, eroding the mortar so that the "bricks" are not secured in their proper place. A variety of outside agents, including detergents, acetone, chlorine, and other chemicals, and even prolonged water immersion can harm the barrier, or the barrier may be deficient for genetic reasons.

The barrier's main components are ceramides, fatty acids, and cholesterol, all different kinds of lipids. These must be present in the right proportion to keep the skin watertight. An impaired barrier will tend toward both dryness and sensitivity. Dryness results when skin moisture evaporates. Sensitivity results when a deficient barrier permits the entry of outside irritants.

Repairing the skin barrier with the right skin care products will help treat a variety of skin conditions. Incorporating key dietary nutrients, such as essential fatty acids and cholesterol, provides the necessary building blocks. Nutrient deficiencies can weaken your skin's ability to repair and rebuild, which is why people who take cholesterol-lowering drugs often have dry skin.

## Oil Production

The skin has many oil (sebaceous) glands, which secrete oil that contains wax esters, triglycerides, and squalene. These fats (or lipids) form a film that helps keep moisture in the skin. While increased sebum production results in oily skin, the opposite is not always the case, as dry skin can also arise from an impaired skin barrier. Oil production can be affected by diet, stress, and hormones—as well as genetics. In a study of twenty pairs each of identical and nonidentical same-sex twins, identical twins had virtually identical amounts of oil production, while the nonidentical twins had significantly different amounts.

Your results on the O/D score portion of the questionnaire will reveal not only which factor is predominant but also, depending on your degree of oiliness and dryness, the skin issues you'll experience and the way you should address them.

## FACTOR TWO: SKIN SENSITIVITY: SENSITIVE VS. RESISTANT

Resistant skin has a solid skin barrier that shields the skin cells, keeping allergens and irritating substances from the deeper skin layers. Unless sunburned, your skin rarely stings, reddens, or develops acne, allowing resistant types to use most products without reacting. However, the irony is that many products may not be potent enough to penetrate the "thick" barrier and deliver results.

Sensitive skin, which is reported by over 40 percent of people, has a weaker barrier, making it vulnerable to many kinds of skin reactions. While many products target sensitive skin, there are four very different subtypes of sensitive skin, so your treatments and products must address your unique subtype:

> **Acne subtype:** Develops acne, blackheads, or whiteheads
> **Rosacea subtype:** Develops recurring flushing, facial redness, and hot sensation
> **Stinging subtype:** Develops stinging or burning of skin
> **Allergic subtype:** Develops redness, itching, and flaking of skin

All of these sensitive skin subtypes have one thing in common: inflammation. That's why all the treatments for "S" types are geared to reduce inflammation and remove its cause.

## Acne Subtype

Between 40 and 50 million Americans are troubled by acne, with eleven- to twenty-five-year-olds accounting for 70 to 80 percent of acne sufferers, while many adult women have acne resulting from hormonal imbalance. Adults are often more perturbed by acne than teens.

Three main factors contribute to acne: increased oil production, clogged pores, and a bacteria called *P. acnes.* Here's how they interact: Oil causes the dead skin cells to stick together, leading to a clogged pore, which is called a blackhead or a whitehead. Bacteria then move into the pore, producing in- flammation, which manifests as redness and pus. Addressing acne requires medications that decrease oil secretion, unclog pores, and kill bacteria. I'll provide recommendations for specific treatments in the prescriptive sec- tions of each type chapter.

## Rosacea Subtype

Affecting tens of millions of Americans, rosacea typically begins in adults over twenty-five years old. Its symptoms are facial redness, flushing, pim- ples, and the formation of prominent blood vessels in the face. Prior to age twenty-five, people prone to rosacea may experience frequent blushing and facial redness with strong emotion. The same bacteria that causes ul- cers *(H. pylori)* may contribute to rosacea, some studies show. Rosacea sufferers with inflammatory bumps and facial redness should be tested for *H. pylori,* which can be treated with oral antibiotics. If you suffer from rosacea, please see your dermatologist for the many effective prescriptive treatments.

## Stinging Subtype

Stinging in response to products and ingredients is not due to allergies, but to more sensitive nerve endings. In dermatology, tests (like the lactic acid stinging test) can determine whether or not you're a "stinger." If you are, you may experience terrible stinging in response to benzoic acid, present in many products such as K-Y Jelly and vaginal yeast infection creams.

Skin stinging is not necessarily accompanied by redness or irritation, al- though it's more common in people who experience facial flushing as well. "Stingers" should avoid products that contain the following ingredients:

Alpha hydroxy acids (glycolic acid)
Benzoic acid
Bronopol
Cinnamic acid compounds
Dowicil 200
Formaldehyde
Lactic acid
Propylene glycol
Quaternary ammonium compounds
Sodium lauryl sulfate
Sorbic acid
Urea
Vitamin C

## Allergic Subtype

When the protective outermost layer of the skin breaks down or weakens, substances can seep around the skin cells and penetrate to deeper layers of the skin. Through these gaps, allergens, chemicals, and other irritants come in from the outside, invading inner levels of the skin tissue and bloodstream, and triggering an inflammatory response. While this is the mechanism for topical skin allergies, there can also be internal allergies to foods or other substances that trigger an inflammatory response expressed via the skin.

A recent epidemiological survey in Great Britain revealed that 23 percent of women and 13.8 percent of men experience an adverse reaction to a personal care product over the course of a year. While stinging is the most common reaction, allergies to cosmetic ingredients also occur. To identify cosmetic ingredient allergies, dermatologists perform patch tests, in which twenty to one hundred ingredients are taped to a person's back. Twenty-four to forty-eight hours later, when the tape is removed, reddened or swollen areas indicate allergies. Up to 10 percent of patients test allergic to at least one cosmetic-product ingredient, according to various studies. But many more may be allergic, as most people don't consult a physician; instead they simply discontinue using the products that bother them.

The most common allergens are fragrances and preservatives. People who use a variety of skin care products are more likely to develop allergies because they have been exposed to more ingredients. People with dry skin (indicating an impaired skin barrier) will tend to have more topical skin allergies. However, whatever your type, due to the high rate of people who experience these allergies, there is no way to be absolutely certain that a given product is right for you, without patch testing. That's why I always recommend that people with sensitive skin try out a product sample, if possible, prior to purchase. If your skin reacts to many ingredients, you may need to consult a dermatologist to identify the specific ones that cause a problem, so you can avoid them.

Allergies are most common in Dry, Sensitive Skin Types, which is why in Chapters Twelve through Fifteen, I'll show how to strengthen the skin barrier to alleviate this problem.

## FACTOR THREE: SKIN PIGMENTATION: PIGMENTED VS. NON-PIGMENTED

The pigmented vs. non-pigmented scale in my questionnaire measures the likelihood of developing unwanted dark spots on the face or chest. Although the test will also take into account skin color and ethnicity, that is not as important in my system as determining the tendency toward unwanted spots. That's why people of all ethnicities can score as any of the sixteen Skin Types. That being said, in some cases, the majority of those with a particular Skin Type may come from certain ethnic backgrounds, while people from a very different ethnicity might be in the minority for that particular type.

Why do I place such emphasis on unwanted dark spots? Twenty-one percent of visits to the dermatologist are for their treatment. Over eighty thousand people annually buy over-the-counter (nonprescription) skin care products to reduce their dark spots. Various kinds of dark spots cause cosmetic concern. In this book, I'll focus on those that are avoidable and removable without surgery. Birthmarks, moles, and scaling patches called seborrheic keratoses are outside of that scope. Instead I'll focus on melasma, sun spots (solar lentigos), and freckles, which can be prevented and treated with skin care products and procedures.

## Dark Spots

**Melasma,** also known as the "mask of pregnancy," consists of light or dark brown or gray patches ranging from the size of a dime to large areas on the face or chest. Appearing in sun-exposed areas, it's more common in pregnant women or those on estrogen therapy, whether birth control pills or hormone replacement. Melasma can be stressful and, in severe cases, even disfiguring. More commonly seen in darker-skinned people, such as Asians, Latin Americans, and African Americans, melasma is difficult to cure but can be controlled with the right skin care products and procedures. Pigmented types with any combination of the other three factors can have melasma.

**Solar lentigos** are caused by sun exposure and sunburns. They're completely preventable with sun avoidance and sun protection. Popping up on people of all skin and hair colors, solar lentigos result from environmental factors, like excess sun, more than genes. I feel that they contribute to the appearance of aging as much or more than wrinkles, a view shared by Asians, who are often more concerned with dark spots than wrinkles.

My patients often tell me that they want "skin like yours," referring to the fact that my complexion is free of spots and wrinkles, both of which contribute to an aged appearance. Yet many people focus more on wrinkles, not recognizing how spots detract from skin's youthfulness. On the first visit, I use a Wood's light (black light) or a UVB camera to reveal facial dark spots before they are visible in ordinary light. Most people are shocked by what they see in the mirror. If you're an Oily, Resistant, Pigmented, and Tight Skin Type (ORPT) with ample solar lentigos, follow the recommendations aimed at wrinkle prevention for Oily, Resistant, Pigmented, and Wrinkled (ORPW) as a preventive. The good news is that my recommendations for products and procedures can make a dramatic difference in the way your skin looks.

**Freckles,** also called ephelides, are associated with red hair and fair skin, while solar lentigos are not, although their appearance is similar. The gene believed to be responsible for freckles is the MC1R gene, which is closely associated with fair skin and red hair. While you can't control your genes, you can control sun exposure. Freckles appear early in childhood, increase as a result of sunburn before the age of twenty, and partly disappear with age, while solar lentigos worsen with age. Because fair-skinned redheads, those most prone to freckles, frequently burn and cannot tan, they often end up avoiding the sun, resulting in less cumulative lifetime sun exposure than people with solar lentigos. However, these fair-skinned redheads are at a higher risk of melanoma, which increases with a history of frequent sunburns and sun exposure.

Unlike people with many solar lentigos, people with freckles can fall into the tight group if they've avoided sun exposure and followed good skin habits, such as eating an antioxidant-rich diet, not smoking, and using retinoids.

## Ethnicity and Skin Tone

While people with a darker skin color are more likely to fall into the pigmented category, not all dark-skinned people are pigmented types, with pigment problems. Those with even skin tones and no spots will be Non-Pigmented Skin Types, even though they have darker-toned skin. On the other hand, light-skinned people who freckle and get melasma or solar lentigos may fall into the P category. The P/N scale measures the tendency to develop unwanted dark spots, not ethnicity.

Skin pigment–producing cells (called melanocytes) produce skin pigment (melanin), which creates skin color as well as all the forms of pigmentation I've mentioned. Skin pigment formation can be prevented by two main mechanisms. The first is to inhibit the enzyme tyrosinase, which prevents the formation of melanin. Many topical cosmetic ingredients such as hydroquinone, kojic acid, arbutin, and licorice extract are tyrosinase inhibitors. The second method of preventing the production of skin color is to forestall the transfer of the color into the skin cells. Studies show that niacinamide and soy prevent that transfer, which is why they are in skin lightening products.

## Pigmentation and Skin Cancer Risk

Pigmentation contributes to your risks of getting the various types of skin cancer, which I'll detail in the specific Skin Types chapters. Melanoma skin cancers result when the pigment cells that produce color become cancerous. Though curable if caught early, this form of cancer can metastasize very rapidly, making early detection essential. Non-melanoma skin cancers are cancers of the skin cells themselves. There are two varieties. Basal cell cancers occur at the basal skin level between the dermis and epidermis. These can be easily removed but may leave scars. Squamous cells grow on the top layer of skin, and although they can metastasize, they are less deadly than melanoma. All should be checked for regularly and treated promptly. Guidelines for detection can be found in "Signs of Melanoma: The A, B, C, and Ds" in Chapter Five, and "How to Recognize a Non-Melanoma Skin Cancer" in Chapter Seven. When in doubt, consult a dermatologist.

## Ultraviolet Light

When UV light hits the skin, it stimulates an increased production of skin pigment, which is what we call tanning. This is the skin's major defense against further UV damage. In addition to tanning skin, ultraviolet light worsens melasma and causes sun spots (solar lentigos). UVB rays cause an immediate sunburn; UVA rays cause long-term damage. Many sunscreens do not block both types of UV light. Even broad-spectrum sunscreens do not block 100 percent of the sun. Sun avoidance is the most important method of preventing skin pigmentation.

Light-skinned people with high P scores are likely to have freckles and may also be at a risk for melanoma. Latin Americans, Asians, and Italians are often on the cusp of the P/N scale.

## FACTOR FOUR: WRINKLED VS. TIGHT

The two main processes of skin aging are intrinsic and extrinsic. Intrinsic aging is your individual genetic programming, which unfolds over time. It's inevitable and beyond your control. Extrinsic aging results from external factors—such as smoking, pollution, poor nutrition, and sun exposure—that can be changed.

Of these, the most universally experienced extrinsic factor is sun exposure, and that's why I place great emphasis on achieving adequate protection. Here I'll overview the basic principles of sun protection, while in the Skin Type chapters, I'll recommend the appropriate products to be employed.

### Daily Sunscreen Use

Make it a habit to apply sunscreen every morning whether you plan to be indoors or out. UVA easily penetrates windows to send harmful sun rays into buildings, cars, and airplanes. Keep your favorite sunblock in your car, desk, and purse in case you forget to apply it as part of your morning routine. Select a product with a minimum SPF of 15 for daily protection, when you will not be receiving prolonged sun exposure. You can also derive sun protection from a variety of skin care products, such as moisturizers, facial foundations, and facial powders that contain SPF. Just make sure that you use a combination of products to assure a combined SPF of at least 15 when they are used together. Never trust a powder or a facial foundation to provide an appropriate SPF. You must use them over a sunscreen or a moisturizing sunscreen to be truly protected.

## Sunscreen Application

To apply, squeeze a quarter-size portion of the product and apply it to your entire face, neck, hands, and chest. Make sure to apply it to all exposed areas that give away your age. (I can almost always tell someone's age by looking at the hands, neck, and chest.) Since there are no procedures that effectively turn back the clock for the neck, it's vital to protect these areas if you want to remain youthful looking.

If you plan to expose the rest of your body to the sun for more than fifteen minutes, apply sunscreen to your legs, shoulders, arms, back, and feet too.

## Increased Sun Exposure

If you swim, play sports, go to the beach, drive on a sunny day, or experience any other form of increased sun exposure, I recommend doing the following:

- Wear a broad-spectrum sunscreen of SPF 45–60 and reapply it every hour.
- Apply your sunscreen thirty minutes prior to sun exposure so it can adequately penetrate the skin.
- Confine your exposure to the times when the sun is less powerful, before ten AM and after four PM.
- Stay under an umbrella when possible.
- Wear protective SPF clothing, available from www.sunprecautions.com and other suppliers.

In addition, apply sunscreen to your body, as clothes provide less protection than most people realize. A normal T-shirt has an SPF of only 5, while tighter weave fabrics offer more protection. You can apply sunscreen to the eye area unless you experience itching, burning, or irritation. In very hot weather, or if you are involved in active sports, you may find that if you sweat, the sunscreen runs into your eyes, causing a burning sensation. If this occurs, look for a sunscreen containing non-stinging ingredients such as titanium dioxide or zinc oxide.

Here's a secret: Sunbathing after prolonged swimming increases your risk for harmful sunburns. Several studies have demonstrated that when exposed to either fresh or salt water, the skin's susceptibility to sunburn increases. But increased sunburn risk does not translate into increased tanning, other studies reveal. So this common practice should be avoided, especially for non-pigmented skin types, who are more susceptible to UV ray damage due to the lack of pigment (melanin), which acts to protect skin from ultraviolet injury.

To enjoy swimming in warm weather while preventing this harmful water-sunburn synergy, after you swim, towel off, apply an ample SPF sunscreen of 30 or more, put on proper clothing, and allow your skin to dry for twenty minutes prior to sun exposure.

## Wrinkle Prevention

While sun protection is key to wrinkle prevention, there are some other factors. The epidermis, or top skin layer, makes the skin look radiant and smooth; wrinkles are caused by changes in the lower layer of the skin, the dermis. Unfortunately, many skin care ingredients cannot penetrate far enough into the dermis to affect wrinkles. But there are a few exceptions. Ingredients like nonprescription retinols and retinoids (obtained via prescription) help to prevent the formation of wrinkles. Antioxidants, when used consistently on the skin, will likely prevent some of the extrinsic aging that occurs. The goal of "wrinkle prevention" is to stop the loss of collagen, elastin, and hyaluronic acid (HA), three important structural components that decrease with age and inflammation. Some antiaging products contain these ingredients and aim to put them "back" into skin, but that is not possible because their molecules are simply too large to be absorbed topically. Although hyaluronic acid added in topical formulas may help hydrate the skin, it does not penetrate and replace lost naturally occurring HA. I wish I had a dollar for every collagen-containing skin cream claiming it would help replace skin collagen and every HA product that claimed it would increase skin HA levels.

Topical agents that stimulate the skin to make its own collagen, elastin, and HA are more effective. Retinoids, vitamin C, and copper peptide have been shown to increase collagen synthesis.

Injecting these components in a cosmetic dermatological procedure called dermal fillers or via a new superficial-level injection called mesotherapy is effective. I'll discuss these options in greater detail later in this book.

If you test out as a Wrinkled Skin Type, don't despair. This is the only Skin Type condition that you can control. Wouldn't you rather know it now and take steps to prevent it? Of course, you cannot control the genetic, or intrinsic, component. However, the extrinsic component is completely under your control.

Sun exposure accelerates the aging process by causing:

- Breakdown of collagen, the supporting structure of the skin
- Breakdown of elastin, which gives skin its resilience and bounce
- Loss of hyaluronic acid, which holds water and gives skin its volume
- Damage to DNA, which can cause cells to go awry, leading to cancer
- Disintegration of enzymes necessary for production of important cell components

The sad fact is that once your skin structures have broken down, it's harder to put them back together again. That's why it's better to protect your skin now, rather than pay later. Avoiding sun exposure, using sunscreen, avoiding cigarette smoke and pollution, taking antioxidant supplements, and eating a diet high in fruits and vegetables can help reduce wrinkling.

In addition, regularly using prescription retinoids and skin care products with antioxidant activity can also help. Experience with patients has suggested to me that Botox injections can prevent wrinkles caused in areas of movement by decreasing movement in those areas. Changing your habits will change you from a W to a T. I am actually a W by nature and a T by choice. If you fall on the boundary between T and W, follow the recommendations for W to help you prevent wrinkles as much as possible.

## HOW THE FOUR FACTORS INTERACT

The way the four factors combine with each other produces certain commonly seen tendencies. For example, Pigmented, Wrinkled Skin Types often have a significant history of sun exposure manifested by wrinkles and solar lentigos. They would do well with retinoids and light treatments. Dry, Sensitive Skin Types have a higher tendency to develop eczema and should use barrier repair moisturizers.

Oily, sensitive types are more likely to develop acne. Lighter-skin OS types, especially those with wrinkles and a strong history of sun damage, have a higher tendency to develop wrinkles and rosacea. Non-Pigmented, Wrinkled Skin Types are more likely to have light skin that wrinkles. Pigmented, tight types most commonly (but not always) have dark skin. Based on Skin Typing as well as these common patterns, my hope is that companies will one day quite soon develop products that focus on your specific needs.

Now it's time to discover your Skin Type by answering the questionnaire in the next chapter. Afterward, you can refer back to this chapter to understand how the science of your predominant factors impacts your skin. Or you may prefer to go directly to your Skin Type chapter.

# CHAPTER THREE

# Discovering Your Skin Type

■

## HOW I DEVELOPED SKIN TYPING AND THE QUESTIONNAIRE

Many people ask me if I can tell their Skin Type at a glance. Having looked at thousands of people's skin, often I can. However, I'm a scientist and I need to be certain. That's why, with my patients, I always double-check by having them answer the questionnaire. Also, in rare instances their answers will reveal something in their history that is not visible to me. This is more likely to occur with young people, whose faces do not yet reveal the results of their skin's genetics, care, and sun exposure.

This questionnaire is truly comprehensive. Despite the short time needed to take it, it reveals more information than would be covered in a typical office visit. As a result, I can spend that valuable time getting to know my patients and their needs, and also providing dermal fillers and other cosmetic treatments. Since everyone's feelings about their face and looks are so personal I like to get to know my patients so that I can address both skin care and their worries, fears, and frustrations about their skin problems. Using this questionnaire gives me more time to do that and still get home to spend time with my two young sons and husband.

Since my patients know that I write a monthly column called "Cosmeceutical Critique" on skin care ingredients in *Skin and Allergy News* (www.skin andallergynews.com), every week a few dozen ask me to devise a specific skin care regimen right for them. And for many years, I did just that. That's how, over time, I saw a pattern emerge, which evolved into my understanding that there are four factors in evaluating people's skin—and as a result, sixteen distinct Skin Types.

To identify my patients' Skin Types, I began asking the questions that evolved over time into the Baumann Skin Type Questionnaire. As my patients used my regimens and recommendations, and we saw their results, I was able to refine these further to assure that they were truly effective for the different Skin Types. In the process, I learned a great deal about which products and ingredients worked always, sometimes, or never, so that within each Skin Type, I could guide people to skin care that met the particular skin issues they experienced.

I further tested every single question with patients to assure that the questions would reveal the right results. In addition, numerous medical colleagues have offered their input as well. So in taking the questionnaire, you can be assured that it will accurately reveal your Skin Type. The questionnaire is constantly being updated as new science develops. The most recent version of the questionnaire can be found at www.skintypesolutions.com. The online version of the questionnaire calculates your score automatically.

## OVERVIEW OF THE QUESTIONNAIRE

The questionnaire is in four parts, with each part offering key questions, which will cumulatively capture where your skin falls on the spectrum of the four factors, between oily and dry, sensitive and resistant, pigmented and nonpigmented, and wrinkled and tight. While some of the factors are familiar to you, some of them may not be. But that's fine. You don't need to understand them to respond. The questions themselves are simple and will prompt you.

In the previous chapter, I explained each of the four factors and the skin characteristics common to both ends of the spectrum within each of the factors. Further information about these factors and how they interact will be revealed in the chapters on the Skin Types.

In taking the test, all you have to do is answer as honestly as you can. Consider it a game. Where I ask you to go without moisturizer and check your skin, or wear foundation but not powder, do it (unless you're a guy)! Of course, you can always guess, but you'll get the most accurate results from following the directions as described. If you haven't really noticed the condition of your skin sufficiently to answer certain questions, take a day or so, and pay attention to how your skin appears, feels, and reacts in the various common situations described, and then go back and retake the test. Unless specifically focused on something in the past, all questions refer to how your skin is now, and should be answered accordingly. Do not leave any questions blank. If necessary, answer *e*, which will be scored as 2.5 points, making it a neutral answer that will not affect the outcome of your total score. You'll get the most accurate Skin Type results if you answer *a*, *b*, *c*, or *d*, so don't pick *e* unless you really can't answer the question.

# Baumann Skin Type Questionnaire

## PART ONE
## OILY VS. DRY

This section measures skin oil production and hydration. Studies show that people's preconceptions about whether their skin is oily or dry are often inaccurate. Don't allow your preconceptions or what others think and say about your skin to bias your answers.

1. After washing your face, don't apply any moisturizer, sunscreen, toner, powder, or other products. Two to three hours later, look in a mirror under bright lights. Your forehead and cheeks feel or appear:
   a. Very rough, flaky, or ashy
   b. Tight
   c. Well hydrated with no reflection of light  K  -3
   d. Shiny with reflection of bright light  M  -4

2. In photos, your face appears shiny:
   a. Never, or you've never noticed shine
   b. Sometimes  K  -2
   c. Frequently
   d. Always  M  -4

3. Two to three hours after applying makeup foundation (also known as base) but no powder, your makeup appears:
   a. Flaky or caked in wrinkles  K  -1
   b. Smooth
   c. Shiny  M  -3
   d. Streaked and shiny
   e. I do not wear facial foundation.

   K  6
   M = 11

4. When in a low-humidity environment, if you don't use moisturizers or sunscreen, your facial skin:
   a. Feels very dry or cracks
   b. Feels tight

c. Feels normal    K - 3
d. Looks shiny, or I never feel that I need moisturizer    M -4
e. Don't know

9   15

5. Look in a magnifying mirror. How many large pores, the size of the end of a pin or greater, do you have?
    a. None
    b. A few in the T-zone (forehead and nose) only    K
    c. Many    M
    d. Tons!
    e. Don't know (Note: Please look again and only answer *e* if you cannot determine this.)

6. You would characterize your facial skin as:
    a. Dry
    b. Normal    K
    c. Combination
    d. Oily    M

7. When you use soap that suds, bubbles, and foams vigorously, your facial skin:
    a. Feels dry or cracks
    b. Feels slightly dry but does not crack
    c. Feels normal    K M
    d. Feels oily
    e. I do not use soap or other foaming cleansers. (If this is because they make your skin dry, pick *a*.)

8. If not moisturized, your facial skin feels tight:
    a. Always
    b. Sometimes
    c. Rarely    M
    d. Never    K

9. You have clogged pores (blackheads or whiteheads):
    a. Never
    b. Rarely
    c. Sometimes    M
    d. Always    K

**10.** Your face is oily in the T-zone (forehead and nose):
    a. Never
    b. Sometimes  K
    c. Frequently
    d. Always  M

**11.** Two to three hours after applying moisturizer your cheeks are:
    a. Very rough, flaky, or ashy
    b. Smooth
    c. Slightly shiny  K
    d. Shiny and slick, or I do not use moisturizer  M

**Scoring of O vs. D:**

Give yourself 1 point for every *a* answer, 2 points for every *b*, 3 points for every *c*, 4 points for every *d*, and 2.5 points for every *e* answer.

Enter your total O/D score here: _____

If your score is between 34–44 you have very oily skin.  39 – M
If your score is between 27–33 you have slightly oily skin.  27 – K
If your score is between 17–26 you have slightly dry skin.
If your score is between 11–16 you have dry skin.

If you scored between 27–44, you are an **O Skin Type.**  – M K
If you scored between 11–26, you are a **D Skin Type.**

## PART TWO
# SENSITIVE VS. RESISTANT

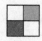

This section measures your skin's tendency to develop pimples, redness, flushing, and itching, all signs of sensitive skin.

**1.** You get red pimples on your face:
    a. Never
    b. Rarely  – M      2
    c. At least once a month
    d. At least once a week  K      4

2. Skin care products (including cleansers, moisturizers, toners, and makeup) cause your face to break out, get a rash, itch, or sting:
   a. Never
   b. Rarely  – M
   c. Often  – K
   d. Always
   e. I don't wear products on my face.

3. Have you ever been diagnosed with acne or rosacea?
   a. No  – M
   b. Friends and acquaintances tell me I have it.
   c. Yes  – K
   d. Yes, a severe case
   e. Unsure

4. If you wear jewelry that is not 14-carat gold, how often do you get a rash?
   a. Never  – M
   b. Rarely
   c. Often
   d. Always  – K
   e. Unsure

5. Sunscreens make your skin itch, burn, break out, or turn red:
   a. Never
   b. Rarely  – M
   c. Often
   d. Always
   e. I never wear sunscreen.  – K

6. Have you ever been diagnosed with atopic dermatitis, eczema, or contact dermatitis (an allergic skin rash)?
   a. No  – M, K
   b. Friends tell me I have it.
   c. Yes
   d. Yes, a severe case
   e. Unsure

7. How often do you get a rash underneath your rings?
   a. Never  – M
   b. Rarely
   c. Often

8 M

6 K

d. Always

e. I do not wear rings. K

8. Fragranced bubble bath, massage oil, or body lotions make your skin break out, itch, or feel dry:
    a. Never
    b. Rarely  —M
    c. Often  - K
    d. Always
    e. I never use these types of products. (Note: Answer *d* if you don't use them because they cause the above-mentioned problems.)

9. Can you use the soap provided in hotels on your body or face without a problem?
    a. Yes
    b. Most of the time, I don't have a problem.  —M
    c. No, my skin itches, turns red, or breaks out.  —
    d. I would not use it. I've had too many problems in the past!  -K
    e. I carry my own, so I'm unsure.

10. Has someone in your family been diagnosed with atopic dermatitis, eczema, asthma, and/or allergies?
    a. No  —M, K
    b. One family member that I know of
    c. Several family members
    d. Many of my family members have dermatitis, eczema, asthma, and/or allergies.
    e. Unsure

11. What occurs if you use scented laundry detergents or static control sheets in the dryer?
    a. My skin is fine.  — M, K
    b. My skin feels slightly dry.         6M
    c. My skin itches.
    d. My skin itches and gets a rash.     9 K
    e. Unsure, or I've never used them

12. How often do your face and/or neck get red after moderate exercise, and/or with stress or a strong emotion, such as anger?
    a. Never
    b. Sometimes

c. Frequently – M,K

d. Always

13. **How often do you tend to get red and flushed after drinking alcohol?**
    a. Never
    b. Sometimes
    c. Frequently
    d. Always, or I don't drink because of this problem
    e. I never drink alcohol. – M,K

14. **How often do you get red and flushed after eating spicy or hot (temperature) foods or beverages?**
    a. Never    – M
    b. Sometimes
    c. Frequently
    d. Always
    e. I never eat spicy food. (Note: If you don't eat spicy or hot food because of facial flushing, pick *d*.)    K

15. **How many visible red or blue broken blood vessels do you have (or did you have prior to treatment) on your face and nose?**
    a. None   –M,K
    b. Few (one to three on entire face, including nose)
    c. Some (four to six on entire face, including nose)
    d. Many (over seven on entire face, including nose)

16. **Your face looks red in photographs:**
    a. Never, or I never noticed it – K
    b. Sometimes   – M
    c. Frequently
    d. Always

17. **People ask you if you are sunburned, even when you are not:**
    a. Never    – M K
    b. Sometimes
    c. Frequently   M
    d. Always
    e. I always *am* sunburned. (You bad thing!)

10·5M

11K

**18.** You get redness, itching, or swelling from makeup, sunscreen, or skin care products:

    a. Never   M

    b. Sometimes K /

    c. Frequently

    d. Always

                                                 1M

                                               2K

    e. I do not use these products. (Note: Answer *d* if you don't use them because of redness, itching, or swelling.)

**Scoring of S vs. R:**

Give yourself 1 point for every *a* answer, 2 points for every *b*, 3 points for every *c*, 4 points for every *d*, and 2.5 for every *e* answer.

Enter your total S/R score here: _____    27.5 M

                                                     42 K

If you've ever received a diagnosis of acne, rosacea, contact dermatitis, or eczema from a dermatologist, add 5 to your score. If another type of physician has diagnosed you with these conditions, add 2 to your score.

If your score is between 34–72 you have very sensitive skin. (Don't worry, I'll help!)

If your score is between 30–33 you have somewhat sensitive skin. Following my recommendations may move you into the R Skin Type.

If your score is between 25–29 you have somewhat resistant skin.

If your score is between 18–24 you have very resistant skin. (Lucky you!)

If you scored between 30–77, you are an **S Skin Type.**   — K

If you scored between 18–29, you are an **R Skin Type.**   ⁻ M

## PART THREE
# PIGMENTED VS. NON-PIGMENTED SKIN

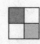

This section measures your skin's tendency to form melanin, a skin pigment that produces darker skin tones as well as dark patches, freckles, and dark areas after trauma. Melanin also helps you tan rather than burn.

1. After you have a pimple or ingrown hair, it's followed by a dark brownish/black spot:
    a. Never or I have not noticed  — K
    b. Sometimes  — M
    c. Frequently
    d. Always
    e. I never get pimples or ingrown hairs.

2. After you cut yourself, how long does the brown (not pink) mark remain?
    a. I don't get a brown mark or I have not noticed.  — M K
    b. A week
    c. A few weeks
    d. Months

3. How many dark patches did you develop on your face when you were pregnant, on birth control pills, or taking hormone replacement therapy (HRT)?
    a. None  — M K
    b. One
    c. A few
    d. A lot
    e. This question does not apply to me (because I am male, or because I have never been pregnant or taken birth control pills or HRT, or because I'm unsure whether I have dark spots). K

4. Do you have any dark patches on your upper lip or cheeks? Or have you had any in the past that you've had removed?
    a. No
    b. I'm not sure.
    c. Yes, they are (or were) slightly noticeable.
    d. Yes, they are (or were) very noticeable.

5. Do the dark patches on your face get worse when you go in the sun?
    a. I have no dark patches.
    b. Unsure
    c. Slightly worse
    d. A lot worse
    e. I wear sunscreen on my face every day and never get sun. (Note: If you use constant sun protection because you're afraid you might get dark patches or freckles, answer d.)

6. Have you been diagnosed with melasma, light or dark brown or gray patches, on your face?
 a. No
 b. Yes, but it went away.
 c. Yes, and I have them now.
 d. Yes, and I have a severe case now.
 e. Unsure

7. Do you have, or have you ever had, small brown spots (freckles or sun spots) on your face, chest, back, or arms?
 a. No
 b. Yes, a few (one to five)
 c. Yes, many (six to fifteen)
 d. Yes, tons (sixteen or more)

8. When exposed to sun for the first time in several months, your skin:
 a. Burns only
 b. Burns, then gets darker
 c. Gets darker
 d. My skin is already dark, so it is hard to see if it gets darker. (You can't pick "I never had sun exposure." Think of childhood experiences!)

9. What happens after you have had many days of consecutive sun exposure:
 a. I sunburn and blister, but my skin does not change color.
 b. My skin becomes slightly darker.
 c. My skin becomes much darker.
 d. My skin is already dark, so it is hard to see if it gets darker.
 e. Unsure (Again, you can't pick "I never had sun." If you really have to pick *e*, first consider all childhood experiences.)

10. What is your natural hair color? (If gray, state color before graying.)
 a. Blond
 b. Brown
 c. Black
 d. Red

11. If you have dark spots on your skin in areas of sun exposure, add 5 points to your score.

**Scoring of P vs. N:**

Give yourself 1 point for every *a* answer, 2 points for every *b*, 3 points for every *c*, 4 points for every *d*, and 2.5 points for every *e* answer.

Enter your total P/N score here: _____

If you scored between 31–45, you are a **P Skin Type.**
If you scored between 10–30, you are an **N Skin Type.** — M,K

## PART FOUR
# WRINKLED VS. TIGHT

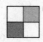

This section measures your tendency to wrinkle, as well as how wrinkled you are right now. Some of my patients confessed that they cheated on this section to come out as a T—*after* I caught them doing it. Don't do that! You're only cheating yourself out of using therapies that could prevent wrinkles. Changing your habits now could change your score in the future from a W to a T. So be honest and get the right treatments if you need them.

1. Do you have facial wrinkles?
    a. No, not even with movement such as smiling, frowning, or lifting my eyebrows.
    b. Only when I move, such as smiling, frowning, or lifting my eyebrows.
    c. Yes, with movement and a few at rest without movement.
    d. Wrinkles are present even if I'm not smiling, frowning, or lifting my brows.

In answering questions 2–7, please respond according to how you would compare yourself and other family members to *all* other ethnic groups, not just your own. For family members whom you may not have known, please ask other family members or refer to photographs, where possible.

**2.** How old does/did your mother's facial skin look?

    a. Five to ten years younger than her age

    b. Her age

    c. Five years older than her age

    d. More than five years older than her age

    e. Not applicable; I was adopted or I cannot remember.

**3.** How old does/did your father's facial skin look?

    a. Five to ten years younger than his age

    b. His age

    c. Five years older than his age

    d. More than five years older than his age

    e. Not applicable; I was adopted or I cannot remember.

**4.** How old does/did your maternal grandmother's facial skin look?

    a. Five to ten years younger than her age

    b. Her age

    c. Five years older than her age

    d. More than five years older than her age

    e. Not applicable; I was adopted, never knew her, or cannot remember.

**5.** How old does/did your maternal grandfather's facial skin look?

    a. Five to ten years younger than his age

    b. His age

    c. Five years older than his age

    d. More than five years older than his age

    e. Not applicable; I was adopted, never knew him, or cannot remember.

**6.** How old does/did your paternal grandmother's facial skin look?

    a. Five to ten years younger than her age

    b. Her age

    c. Five years older than her age

    d. More than five years older than her age

    e. Not applicable; I was adopted, never knew her, or cannot remember.

**7.** How old does/did your paternal grandfather's facial skin look?

    a. Five to ten years younger than his age

    b. His age

    c. Five years older than his age

    d. More than five years older than his age

    e. Not applicable; I was adopted, never knew him, or cannot remember.

8. At any time in your life, have you ever tanned your skin on an ongoing basis for more than two weeks per year? If so, for how many total years did you do this? Please count tanning from playing tennis, fishing, playing golf, skiing, or other outdoor activities. The beach is not the only place you can get a tan.
    a. Never
    b. One to five years
    c. Five to ten years
    d. More than ten years

9. At any time in your life, have you ever engaged in seasonal tanning of two weeks per year or less? (Yes, summer vacation counts!) If so, how often?
    a. Never
    b. One to five years
    c. Five to ten years
    d. More than ten years

10. Based on the places you've lived, how much daily sun exposure have you received in your life?
    a. Little; I've mostly lived in places that are gray and overcast.
    b. Some; I've lived in less sunny climes at times, but also in places with more regular sun.
    c. Moderate; I've lived in places with a fair amount of sun exposure.
    d. A lot; I've lived in tropical, Southern, or very sunny locales.

11. How old do you think you look?
    a. One to five years younger than your age
    b. Your age
    c. Five years older than your age
    d. More than five years older than your age

12. During the last five years, how often have you allowed your skin to tan either intentionally or unintentionally through outdoor sports or other activities?
    a. Never
    b. Once a month
    c. Once a week
    d. Daily

13. How often, if ever, have you been to a tanning bed?
    a. Never

      b. One to five times

      c. Five to ten times

      d. Many times

**14.** Over your entire life, how many cigarettes have you smoked (or been exposed to)?

      a. None

      b. A few packs

      c. Several to many packs

      d. I smoke every day.

      e. I've never smoked but I've lived with, been raised by, or worked with people who regularly smoked in my presence.

**15.** Please describe the air pollution where you reside:

      a. The air is fresh and clean.

      b. For part of the year, but not all of the year, I reside in a place with clean air.

      c. The air is slightly polluted.

      d. The air is very polluted.

**16.** Please describe the length of time that you have used retinoid facial creams such as retinol, Renova, Retin-A, Tazorac, Differin, or Avage:

      a. Many years

      b. Occasionally

      c. Once for acne when I was younger

      d. Never

**17.** How often do you currently eat fruits and vegetables?

      a. At every meal

      b. Once a day

      c. Occasionally

      d. Never

**18.** Over your lifetime, what percentage of your daily diet has consisted of fruits and vegetables? (Note: Don't count juices unless they are freshly squeezed.)

      a. 75–100 percent

      b. 25–75 percent

      c. 10–25 percent

      d. 0–10 percent

19. What is your natural skin color (without tanning or self-tanners)?
    a. Dark
    b. Medium
    c. Light
    d. Very light

20. What is your ethnicity? (Please choose the best answer.)
    a. African American/Caribbean/Black
    b. Asian/Indian/Mediterranean/Other
    c. Latin American/Hispanic
    d. Caucasian

21. If you are sixty-five or older, add 5 points to your score.

**Scoring of W vs. T:**

Give yourself 1 point for every *a* answer, 2 points for every *b*, 3 points for every *c*, 4 points for every *d*, and 2.5 points for every *e* answer.

Enter your total W/T score here: _____

If you scored between 41 and 85, you are a **W Skin Type.**
If you scored between 20 and 40, you are a **T Skin Type.**

To define your final Skin Type results, please take all the factor indications that you have scored (in the order of your test responses) and write them in here:

My O/D score is _____, which equals _____.

My S/R score is _____, which equals _____.

My P/N score is _____, which equals _____.

My W/T score is _____, which equals _____.

Put them together and now you know your Skin Type! If you are confused about your skin type, visit www.skintypesolutions.com and take the online quiz, which will automatically calculate your score. The online quiz has photographs to assist with your answer selections.

In this edition of the book, your Baumann Skin Type has been assigned a number from 1 to 16 in order to help you easily remember your skin type. We all remember things in different ways. You can remember your Baumann Skin Type in three ways—whichever is easier for you: 1) by the corresponding letters such as OSPW, or 2) by a number between 1 and 16, or 3) by a color. The Baumann Skin Type colors and number key can be found at www.BaumannSkinTypes.com.

## WHAT YOUR TEST REVEALS

Now that you know your Skin Type, you may want to go back and reread the previous chapter, so that you understand where your skin's characteristics place you in each of the four factors. Next, you can turn to your Skin Type chapter and learn all that you need to know about caring for your skin. Here I'll go a little further into your results to explain more about your skin.

## YOUR OILY VS. DRY SCORE

**If your O score is 11–16, you have very dry skin.**

With very dry skin, you may be deficient in natural moisturizing factor (NMF), which is decreased by exposure to UVA light; avoiding sun exposure may help. If your skin is both dry *and* resistant, you may lack NMF, which cannot be replaced.

Hyaluronic acid (HA), which holds skin moisture, decreases with age. People who are dry *and* wrinkled may have less HA.

If you have dry skin, small pores, and minimal acne, you may have decreased oil secretion. Oil production decreases with age (and menopause) and is most common with the Dry, Resistant (DR) Skin Type.

With dry skin, if you suffer from frequent redness and itching, you may have a damaged skin barrier. In this category, you've a higher risk for rashes and eczema, which may run in your family.

**With a score of 17–26, you have slightly dry skin.**

Your Oily/Dry score and your Sensitive/Resistant score can interact. If you score 30 or greater on the S/R scale, you may suffer from *occasional* skin itching, flaking, and redness, indicating a less than perfect skin barrier. The recommendations I'll offer in the chapters for dry, resistant skin will help tackle this range of issues.

If you score less than 25 on the S/R questionnaire, then you probably have an intact skin barrier. Your skin dryness is more likely due to lower levels of natural moisturizing factor (NMF) and/or sebum.

**With a score of 27–33, you have slightly oily skin.**

If your S/R score is 30 or below, you have the ideal degree of skin hydration. You likely have an intact skin barrier, good NMF levels, and enough sebum secretion without having too much to cause such problems as acne. However, if you score 34 or above on the S/R scale, you probably suffer from acne or rosacea.

**With an O/D score over 34, you have very oily skin.**

If you score 30 or below on the S/R scale, you suffer from skin oiliness but only rarely acne, and usually during times of stress or hormonal fluctuations. If so, figuring out what triggers the acne will help you address it.

However, if you score 34 or above on the S/R scale, you probably suffer from acne or rosacea. Your skin's oiliness will help you tolerate products that the drier S types cannot use. The OS chapters will offer recommendations.

## YOUR SENSITIVE VS. RESISTANT SCORE

**With an S/R score over 34,** you are very likely to experience the more severe problems of one or more of the sensitivity subtypes described in Chapter Two.

**With a score of 25–33,** you are likely to experience some problems typical of several of the sensitivity subtypes, or have significant problems within one subtype.

**With a score of 24 or less,** you rarely suffer from the skin sensitivities detailed in Chapter Two. Even if you have a low S/R score, and are a Resistant Skin Type, you still may have occasional acne breakouts or redness; however, they're not the norm. If that occurs, temporarily follow the recommendations for your corresponding Sensitive Skin Type. For example, if you're usually a DRNW but as a result of recent stress, you develop acne, follow the recommendations in the DSNW chapter until your skin returns to its usual state.

I'll not go further into your scoring in the categories of pigmented vs. non-pigmented and wrinkled vs. tight, because your treatment needs and options for skin problems arising from these factors will depend on the issues you actually experience.

## The Skin Type Chapters

While your chapter will contain all the essential information you'll need, you may also find related information in the chapters of Skin Types that are similar, though slightly different, from yours. So if you'd like to know a little more, you can read these related chapters as well. Still you may find additional stories or scientific information that also applies to your Skin Type elsewhere in the book.

Which types are closest to yours? For starters, if you're an OSPT, then an OSPW would be pretty close to you—except that you would not be concerned with wrinkling. People with oily, sensitive skin share common problems, as do people with dry, resistant skin, so if you have the time and interest, you could read those related Skin Type chapters.

If you scored very near the changeover number between the two sides of the spectrum in any of the categories, you might choose to read both types. For example, people who score between 26 and 28 on the Oily/Dry questions have combination skin. While I provide options for combination skin in both the Oily and Dry Skin Type chapters, if you scored a 27 and were an ORPT, you might want to read DRPT as well, since you're pretty close.

For example, let's say that you have scored as an OSNW type, but are borderline dry. You have no problem with skin dryness—until the winter. At that time, you could follow the recommendations for the most similar Dry Skin Type, DSNW, switching back to your original type's regimen and products when warm weather returns. On the other hand, suppose you moved to a very dry climate. In that case, ongoing drying conditions could result in your turning permanently into a Dry Skin Type. To prevent that, read the related dry type chapter and take the precautions recommended to preserve your skin's moisture.

Here's another example: You may be an R type who has never experienced acne or skin rashes—until a stressful situation occurs. That stressful situation can make your skin *behave* like an S type. If that happens, follow the recommendations for your related Sensitive Skin Type, to calm your sensitivity and reduce your stress.

The category of pigmentation is primarily genetic. But if you were borderline between N and P, with a score between 22 and 26, and you are concerned about dark spots, you can follow the P recommendations for preventing and treating them.

Finally, many environmental influences impact people's T/W scores. If you're a tight type, such as a DRPT, but are close to the borderline for wrinkled, you could follow the recommendations for your corresponding wrinkled type, DRPW. That way, you can do everything right to help your skin preserve its tightness.

Now that you know your Skin Type, you can go directly to your Skin Type chapter. There you'll find everything you need to care for your skin with the certainty that when it comes to product choices and treatments, you've finally got it right.

## PART TWO

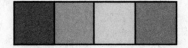

# Skin Care for Oily, Sensitive Skin

# CHAPTER FOUR

# Oily, Sensitive, Pigmented, and Wrinkled: OSPW

## BAUMANN SKIN TYPE NUMBER 7

*"My oily sensitive skin makes it hard to find a daily facial sunscreen. I admit I have not always been good about protecting my skin from the sun and I want to know how to take better care of it. Preventing skin aging is important to me."*

### ABOUT YOUR SKIN

Many people with an Oily, Sensitive, Pigmented, and Wrinkled Skin Type were the first ones on the beach in the morning and the last ones off it at sundown. The envy of all the other types, OSPWs tan to a perfect bronze. You once were the surfer guys, the beach bunnies, the jet-setting socialites with the permanent tan, and the ever-bronzed CEOs. And let's not forget the bikini (or mono-kini) clad Frenchwomen who bake on the beach at Cannes, St. Tropez, and St. Bart's. You are all OSPWs and I see a lot of you in my Miami office when you fly in before (or after) your sun-filled Caribbean vacation.

Unlike non-pigmented folks, who don't tan very well, your pigmented skin turns to gold. And unlike many resistant types who prize their flawless complexions and flee the sun, you once believed that there's nothing like an overall tan to diminish the appearance of the many tiny imperfections, including pimples, acne scars, brown spots, freckles, and other minor blemishes to which your type is prone. A tan shifts attention from blemished to shapely legs. But it's a myth that the sun helps control acne. In fact, studies show that sun exposure increases breakouts by intensifying oil production.

If the questionnaire revealed you as an OSPW but you are *not* a sun worshipper, congratulations for changing your ways or not falling into the routine of sun exposure that most OSPWs follow. Many OSPWs stop getting sun exposure in their adult years but they are left with many skin issues such as wrinkles and brown patches from the previous years of sun.

## SUN EXPOSURE: THE BAD NEWS

I see OSPWs at every stage of the lifespan, and I can testify that the very same golden tan that makes you look great in youth is going to turn you into a dried-up prune as you age. Every day, younger OSPWs parade through my office, convinced that the sun is good for them, and I always wish I could let them eavesdrop on my visits with older OSPWs as they despair over wrinkles, sags, and other signs of aging, frequently forking over a small fortune to make things look right. It's much better to minimize, or at least moderate, your sun exposure now, to avoid paying such a steep price later. What's more, you run the risk of paying an even steeper price than premature aging.

Melanoma is very definitely a risk factor for your Skin Type. Dermatologists take all melanomas extremely seriously, and we're trained to recognize them. Please turn to "Signs of Melanoma: The A, B, C, and D" in Chapter Five and "How to Recognize a Non-Melanoma Skin Cancer" in Chapter Seven for an explanation of how to spot the different kinds of skin cancer. When in doubt, consult a dermatologist.

## AGING AND YOUR SKIN: GETTING REAL

Although genes govern a lot about your Skin Type, when it comes to wrinkling, genetic tendencies interact with lifestyle choices to determine whether your skin is wrinkled or tight. For example, a patient of mine named Janet has dark-toned, oily, resistant, thick skin that is much less prone to wrinkle than that of my former nurse Lisa, who has light, tissue-fine, dry, and sensitive skin. Beyond genetic givens like their physical differences, people can increase or decrease their skin's native tendency through behavior and lifestyle.

Protect your skin and consume antioxidants, and you'll get the best from your skin. Do the opposite, and you'll wind up in my office. When Janet baked in the sun year after year, she lowered the impact of her "good" genes, even though they had kept both her mother and grandmother wrinkle-free into their eighties. On the other hand, Lisa, who regularly wore sunscreen and cared properly for her skin, aged much better than her chain-smoking mother.

That's why, if you fall into this category, it's very likely that your behavior is the prime cause of your skin's wrinkling. However, a small percentage will fall into this category due to genetics. In either case, follow my recommendations to care for and protect your skin.


## A CLOSE-UP LOOK AT YOUR SKIN

If your questionnaire results reveal you to be an OSPW, you may experience any of the following:

- Signs of sun damage
- Red or brown patches
- Areas with dappled brown and white pigment
- Skin spottiness on chest and face
- "Fisherman's face" with broken facial capillaries
- Frequent acne breakouts
- Redness, stinging, and burning in response to many skin care products
- Sunscreens feel oily and make your face appear shiny.
- Regular makeup wears off too easily but ColorStay and other long-lasting makeup brands cause skin redness and itching.
- Wrinkles begin in the late twenties or early thirties.
- Dark spots in areas of trauma such as cuts, burns, bruises, scrapes, and breakouts
- Dark patches on cheeks
- Lipstick bleeds through edges of lips.
- Dark circles under the eyes

Your skin's oiliness can lead to acne, with breakouts triggering pigmentation. Acne scars can often result. For most OSPWs, higher levels of pigment increase the risk of developing unsightly dark spots, which spring up suddenly and take awhile (if ever) to improve. Beyond pimples, many other minor skin irritants can stimulate the production of brown spots, including inflammation, wounds, nicks, and cuts. Hormonal shifts arising from oral contraceptive use and pregnancy can raise estrogen levels, also contributing to brown spots. In addition, sun exposure accelerates your skin's natural tendency to produce the pigment that creates dark spots, sun spots, and freckles.

In fact, nearly all of the symptoms OSPWs typically experience are worsened by sun exposure. Yet due to your skin's sensitivity, it can be hard to find a sunscreen that does not cause burning or redness.

Although I advise against sunbathing, moderate- to darker-skinned

OSPWs usually tan well, with minimal sunburn. Frequent sun exposure can cause a natural buildup of melanin, the pigmenting factor in the skin. Although this contributes to aging and the formation of brown spots, and is therefore not advisable, there is one benefit. Pigmented cells surround the cellular DNA, protecting it from degrading into cancerous cells. Because of the dark-skinned OSPWs' ability to form pigment, this type may be less likely to develop non-melanoma skin cancers.

Are any levels of sun exposure safe? Even if you wear a broad-spectrum sunscreen of SPF 15 or more as I recommend, some minimal sun exposure will occur. That's why to assure you are protected, please follow my advice for sun protection in "Daily Sunscreen Use" in Chapter Two.

## ANTIAGING MYTHS

Because of skin wrinkles, often OSPWs want to use antiaging creams, but many contain ingredients too intense for your sensitive skin. Others are simply not that effective. Many bestselling creams contain hyaluronic acid (HA), a sugar found in the skin that decreases with aging and sun exposure, causing skin to lose its volume. In fact, a highly popular cosmetic dermatological treatment (that I perform on a near daily basis) involves injecting hyaluronic acid to plump up facial wrinkles and sags.

That's why people assume that a cream with HA would deliver the same benefits. But as I explained on page 23, it doesn't, since hyaluronic acid cannot be absorbed into the skin from a cream. Since hyaluronic acid helps hydrate the skin by holding water, applying it via a cream on the outer layer of the skin may actually be counterproductive because in a low-humidity environment it draws water from the skin and dries the skin out. Even people with oily skin, like OSPWs, won't benefit from dehydrating their skin. Reducing oil that causes acne and reducing water that gives the skin its volume are two different things.

You may also be tempted by popular antiaging creams or other skin care products that contain alpha lipoic acid and DMAE (dimethylaminoethanol). While these ingredients can be effective in treating wrinkles for resistant types, sensitive types often don't tolerate them well.

Since antiwrinkle creams can cost as much as $400 for a tiny jar, I can't stress enough how important it is to be aware of exactly what you're allowing to contact your sensitive skin. Fortunately, certain antiaging ingredients really work for you, such as salicylic acid (SA), which decreases skin sensitivity, oiliness, and wrinkles. In addition, products containing nonprescription retinol or a prescription retinoid are great for both minimizing and preventing wrinkles. My recommended products contain these ingredients and will deliver them in your daily regimen.

## THE SENSITIVE SKIN DILEMMA

Extreme skin problems, like wrinkling and dark spots, seem to call for powerful measures, so many OSPWs purchase and try products with strong ingredients, only to find their sensitive skin will not tolerate them. Many OSPWs have trouble finding a sunscreen that they can use without redness or irritation. Skin lighteners that contain bleaching ingredients commonly cause reactions as well.

In the next section of this chapter, I'll teach you how to work with your skin's sensitivity. I'll offer a skin care routine that protects your skin from sun exposure while treating brown spots and wrinkling with products you can safely use. You need ingredients that calm rather than inflame your skin. Learn to recognize and avoid ingredients too irritating for you.

Decrease the reactive combination of oiliness, sensitivity, and pigmentation (preventing breakouts and brown spots) by first avoiding sun exposure and, second, following the protocols I'll offer in the next section of this chapter.

In midlife, after menopause, both oil production and hormonal levels naturally decrease. This change provides relief for many of the skin problems you suffer in youth. However, since your skin tends to wrinkle, the aging process is not that kind to you. That's why I will offer wrinkle prevention strategies you can use when wrinkles start to appear in your twenties and thirties. In addition, you're a good candidate for the advanced skin prescription medications and procedures used to minimize the visible signs of aging.

**Dr. Baumann's Bottom Line:** Protect your skin and treat wrinkles and dark spots as early as possible.

## EVERYDAY CARE FOR YOUR SKIN

The goal of your skin care routine is to address oiliness, brown spots, and wrinkles with products that deliver antioxidant and anti-inflammatory ingredients.

In addition, your daily regimen will also help to address your other skin concerns by preventing and treating both pimples and inflammation.

Anything strong enough to help your wrinkles and dark spots may irritate your skin. I'll recommend products that are strong enough to have an effect while containing antioxidant ingredients (like green tea) and anti-inflammatory ingredients (like licochalone) that both protect your skin and calm its sensitivity. Although wrinkles are your number-one skin problem, dark spots come in a close second. For that reason, I'll provide a two-stage protocol. In the first stage, outlined here, you'll undertake a foundation regimen that will show immediate results in lessening brown spots. Please look over your regimen and then you can select the products you'll need from those I recommend in each category later in this chapter.

If, after two weeks to two months on this regimen, you need further help, I recommend you consult a dermatologist who can offer prescription medications and procedures.

## DAILY SKIN CARE

### REGIMEN FOR REDNESS AND/OR DARK SPOTS:

**AM**

Step 1: Wash with a cleanser

Step 2: Apply a skin lightener

Step 3: Apply eye cream (optional)

Step 4: Apply SPF facial lotion or sunscreen regimen

Step 5: Apply foundation with SPF

Step 6: Apply oil-absorbing powder

**PM**

Step 1: Wash with same cleanser used in AM

Step 2: Apply a skin lightener (optional)

Step 3: Apply a retinol-containing product for dark spots and acne, or a serum for redness and irritation

Step 4: Apply eye cream (optional)

Step 5: Apply moisturizer (optional)

In the morning, clean your face with a cleanser containing salicylic acid (SA) to decrease acne and clean pores while easing pigmentation problems without irritating your sensitive skin. Or if skin is red and inflamed, use a nonfoaming gentle cleanser without salicylic acid. Use a soft washcloth and avoid vigorous rubbing. Next, for brown spots, apply a skin lightener to your entire face. If you suffer predominantly from acne rather than skin redness and irritation, or if you have a lower S/R score (25–30), you can mix your skin lightener with a vitamin C powder, such as Philosophy Hope and a Prayer vitamin C powder. For application instructions, see below. Then you can use an eye cream, if you'd like to. If you have facial redness, you should not use either toners or skin lighteners that contain hydroquinone and vitamin C. Instead choose one with kojic acid and arbutin, such as Philosophy A Pigment of Your Imagination. For redness, you can also add a facial lotion. Next, apply sunscreen. Although an SPF-containing lotion is best for sun protection, sometimes people with very sensitive skin can be allergic to certain sunscreen ingredients. If you experience sensitivity to sunscreens, look for products that contain z-cote, such as SkinCeuticals Sheer Physical UV Defense SPF 50. Finish with makeup foundation and facial powder, if desired.

In the evening, cleanse and remove all makeup with a recommended cleanser. Next, for acne and dark spots, in your hand mix a pea-size portion of the same skin lightener used in the morning with the retinol product (Steps 2 and 3) and apply them together. The retinol product should be applied only in the evening, and will help control acne and dark spots while preventing wrinkles. If you have facial redness, apply the skin lightener to dark spots only. Next, cover the entire face and neck with a serum such as Olay Regenerist Daily Regenerating Serum (Fragrance Free) and follow with a retinol-containing product. If you wish, you can apply an eye cream to the eye area and a light moisturizer to dry skin areas.

## Using Vitamin C Powder

Vitamin C can help to prevent both pigmentation and wrinkles. Philosophy Hope and a Prayer vitamin C powder contains a scoop you can use to pour powder into the palm of your hand along with a dime-size portion of skin lightener. Mix and apply. If you suffer from redness and facial flushing or have a high S/R score (34 or greater), eliminate this product and follow the rest of the morning regimen.

# Choosing and Using Cleansers

When removing makeup, use a nonirritating cleanser containing ingredients such as salicylic acid (SA), aloe vera, licochalone, feverfew, chamomile, or niacinamide, which will reduce redness, inflammation, and acne and help to unclog pores.

## RECOMMENDED CLEANSING PRODUCTS

$ Aveeno Clear Complexion Foaming Cleanser (SA)
$ L'Oréal Advanced RevitaLift Radiant Smoothing Cream Cleanser (SA)
$ Clean & Clear Continuous Control Acne Wash (SA)
$ Eucerin Redness Relief Soothing Cleanser
$ Neutrogena Oil-Free Acne Wash, Redness Soothing Facial Cleanser
$$ Josie Maran Bear Naked Wipes
$$$ Sundari Gentle Gel Cleanser
$$ Paula's Choice Hydralight One Step Face Cleanser
$$ Topix Gly Sal 5-2 Cleanser
$$$ Vivite Exfoliating Facial Cleanser

**Baumann's Choice:** Neutrogena Oil-Free Acne Wash, Redness Soothing Facial Cleanser

If acne is your main problem, and you're free from burning and stinging, you can also use PanOxyl Bar 10% by Stiefel Laboratories.

# Toner Use

Although toners are unnecessary for you, some oily types enjoy their refreshing feeling. You can use a toner after cleansing. If you wish to add this extra step, you can benefit from the anti-inflammatory and pigment- and oil-control ingredients in the recommended toners. However, if you have either a high S/R score (34 or greater) or dry or combination skin (an O/D score of 27 to 35), don't use toners. Also, if any skin products cause redness or stinging, avoid them.

## RECOMMENDED TONERS

$  Burt's Bees Natural Acne Solutions Clarifying Toner
$$  Citrix Antioxidant Toner by Topix
$$  Clinique Acne Solutions Clarifying Lotion
$  Neutrogena Oil-Free Acne Stress Control Triple-Action Toner
$$  Bliss No 'Zit' Sherlock Purifying Cleanser & Toner

**Baumann's Choice:** Burt's Bees Natural Acne Solutions Clarifying Toner

## Pimples

Above all, don't steam your face, apply a hot washcloth, or place an ice cube on a pimple. All of these actions cause rapid changes in temperature, which is strictly a no-no for types prone to inflammation—and that means you. As previously discussed, some people believe that sun exposure will help clear up acne, but since acne typically worsens in summer, I don't believe that it's helpful. The products in your daily regimen should help prevent pimples and acne and, in addition, you can treat breakouts with some of the blemish medications listed below.

If you like, these products can be added to concealer to both treat and cover blemishes. Directly after cleansing or toner application, mix the concealer (in an amount equivalent to one third the size of a pea) with medication and apply to the pimple. Other treatment products or moisturizers should only be applied afterward.

## RECOMMENDED SPOT TREATMENTS FOR PIMPLES

$  Clearasil Daily Acne Control Vanishing Acne Treatment Cream
$  Neutrogena On-the-Spot Acne Treatment, Vanishing Formula
$$  Paula's Choice Clear Extra Strength Acne Fighting Treatment
$$  Proactive Advanced Blemish
$$$  Kinerase Clear Blemish Dissolver
$$  Vichy Laboratories Normaderm Anti-Blemish Intensive Treatment Cream
$$$  Philosophy Hope in a Bottle or On a Clear Day $H_2O_2$

**Baumann's Choice:** Kinerase Clear Blemish Dissolver

# Treating Dark Spots

Apply skin-lightening products to your dark spots only after cleansing and toning but before applying other recommended products. The products listed below should be used as soon as the dark spot appears, and until the spot has completely disappeared. If you find that over-the-counter remedies don't work, speak with your dermatologist about prescription lighteners.

## RECOMMENDED NONPRESCRIPTION SKIN LIGHTENERS

$ Specific Beauy Skin Brightening Serum
$ Skineffects by Dr. Jeffrey Dover Advanced Brightening Complex
$$ PCA Skin Pigment Gel
$$ Paula's Choice Resist Clearly Remarkable Skin Lightening Gel with 2% BHA
$$ Proactive Solution Skin Lightening Lotion
$$ Murad Age Spot & Pigment Lightening Gel
$$ Clinique Even Better Clinical Dark Spot Corrector
$$$ La Roche-Posay Mela-D Dark Spots HQ Free, SPF 15
$$$ Dr. Brandt Flaws No More Lightening Serum
$$$ Vivite Vibrance Therapy

**Baumann's Choice:** Paula's Choice Resist Clearly Remarkable Skin Lightening Gel with 2% BHA because it contains acne fighting BHA as well as skin lighteners

# Moisturizers and Serums

Moisturizers are unnecessary for most oily types; however, if you have a lower O/D score (27–32), feel free to use my recommended moisturizers on dry facial areas. Serums are another option. They often contain healing ingredients in high concentrations, which results in better skin penetration. Contained in a dropper-style bottle, serums are thicker in texture than other products, so a little goes a long way. Use only a few drops and spread over your face as indicated in the regimen. You can apply a moisturizer over the serum if you wish.

When using a retinol or retinoid product, light moisturizing can help offset the flaking that may accompany its use and is helpful if you tested slightly lower on oiliness, from 24 to 30 on the O/D Score.

## RECOMMENDED MOISTURIZERS

- $ CeraVe PM Moisturizing Lotion
- $ Aveeno Positively Radiant Daily Moisturizer SPF 15 or 30
- $ Aveeno Clear Complexion Daily Moisturizer
- $ Neutrogena Oil Free Moisturizer for Sensitive Skin
- $$ Dr. Dennis Gross Skincare Trifix Acne Clearing Lotion
- $$ Canyon Ranch Balance Light-Weight Moisture
- $$ Clinique Even Better Skin Tone Correcting Moisturizer SPF 20
- $$ Vivite Daily Facial Moisturizer SPF 30

**Baumann's Choice:** Aveeno Clear Complexion Daily Moisturizer because its has Total Soy Complex and salicylic acid to prevent acne and brown spots

## RECOMMENDED SERUMS

- $ Olay Regenerist Daily Regenerating Serum (Fragrance Free)
- $ Aveeno Positively Ageless Rejuvenating Serum
- $$ Replenix CF Serum
- $$ Dr. Andrew Weil for Origins Plantidote Mega-Mushroom Face Serum
- $$ Josie Maran Argan Oil
- $$ La Roche-Posay Toleriane Facial
- $$ SkinCeuticals Serum 15

**Baumann's Choice:** Josie Maran Argan Oil because it contains a high concentration of total soy

## RECOMMENDED RETINOL-CONTAINING PRODUCTS

- $ RoC Retinol Correxion Deep Wrinkle Night Cream
- $$ Afirm 2x
- $$ PCA Skin Phase 23 A&C Synergy Serum
- $$ Philosophy Help Me
- $$ Topix Replenix Retinol Smoothing Serum 5x
- $$ Skinceuticals Retinol 0.5

**Baumann's Choice:** Topix Replenix Retinol Smoothing Serum 5x because it also has green tea

## Eye Creams

For dark circles under eyes, use eye creams (like Quintessence Clarifying Under-Eye Serum) that contain retinol and vitamin K to address the blood congestion that causes them. If, after consulting your dermatologist, you choose to use a prescription retinoid around the eye area, dilute it by mixing it with an equal amount of moisturizer.

### RECOMMENDED EYE CREAMS

- $ Boots No7 Time-Resisting Day and Night Eye Care
- $ RoC Eye Cream
- $$ Relastin Eye Silk
- $$ Laura Mercier Eyedration
- $$ Quintessence Clarifying Under-Eye Serum
- $$$ Aveeno Active Naturals Ageless Vitality Elasticity Recharging System, Eye
- $$$ Dr. Brandt Lineless Eye Cream

**Baumann's Choice:** Boots No7 Time-Resisting Day and Night Eye Care

## Masks

Because they deliver concentrated ingredients to your skin for an extended time period, masks can be beneficial. Once or twice a week apply a mask with exfoliating and depigmenting properties, such as MD Formulations Vit-A-Plus Clearing Complex Mask. You can use it in the evening, immediately after cleansing. Follow the instructions on the package, and once you have rinsed it off, you can proceed to Step 2 (applying skin lightener). Or go to a spa or salon for a mask treatment by a spa therapist, making sure to ask for masks for sensitive skin with the depigmenting and anti-inflammatory ingredients I recommend.

## Exfoliation

OSPW skin benefits from nonprescription retinols and prescription retinoid use. And though retinoids can cause flaking, they don't cause dryness. Instead, the flakes signify beneficial skin exfoliation, a process that helps your skin slough off dead cells.

## SHOPPING FOR PRODUCTS

By reading labels, you can also widen your choice of products, selecting those that contain beneficial ingredients for your type while avoiding ones that increase allergic reactions, stinging, burning, redness, acne, inflammation, or oiliness. Take the list below with you when you go shopping so that you can read labels, identify the common culprits, and avoid products containing them. If you have acne or sunscreen sensitivity, double-check labels for ingredients to avoid. Some products on this list may contain ingredients that are not good for those types, but remember: Not everyone reading this chapter has acne or sunscreen sensitivity. If you find additional products beyond the ones I recommend, please tell us at www.skintypesolutions.com so that you can share your find with others of your Skin Type.

Each person with sensitive skin reacts to different ingredients, so selectively test products with suspicious ingredients, and notice how your skin responds. If possible, try products at a beauty counter or obtain samples before you purchase them to make sure that they work for you. As not every reaction is instantaneous, allow twenty-four hours to pass before making your decision. Making that extra effort will save you money and help you treat your skin right.

---

### SKIN CARE INGREDIENTS TO USE

#### To lessen acne:

- Benzoyl peroxide
- Retinol
- Salicylic acid (beta hydroxy acid, or BHA)
- Tea tree oil
- Zinc

#### To reduce inflammation:

- Aloe vera
- Arnica
- Calendula
- Chamomile
- Colloidal oatmeal
- Cucumber
- Dexpanthenol (provitamin B$_5$)
- *Epilobium*
- Feverfew
- Green tea
- Licochalone
- Perilla leaf extract
- Pycnogenol (a pine bark extract)
- Red algae
- Thyme

angustifolium
(willow herb)
- Evening primrose oil

- *Trifolium pretense* (red clover)
- Zinc

### To prevent or lighten dark spots:

- Arbutin
- Bearberry extract
- Cucumber
- *Glycyrrhiza glabra* (licorice extract)

- Hydroquinone
- Mulberry extract
- Niacinamide

### To prevent wrinkles:

- Alpha lipoic acid
- Basil
- Caffeine
- Carrot extract
- Coenzyme $Q_{10}$
- Copper peptide
- Cucumber
- Curcumin (tetrahydracurcumin or turmeric)
- Ferulic acid
- Feverfew
- Ginger
- Ginseng

- Grape seed extract
- Green tea, white tea
- Idebenone
- Lutein
- Lycopene
- Pomegranate
- Pycnogenol (a pine bark extract)
- Rosemary
- Silymarin
- *Trifolium pretense, fabaceae* (red clover)
- Yucca

## SKIN CARE INGREDIENTS TO AVOID

### If you are acne prone:

- Cinnamon oil
- Cocoa butter
- *Cocos nucifera* (coconut oil)
- Isopropyl isostearate

- Isopropyl myristate
- Peppermint oil
- Sodium laurel sulfate

## Sun Protection for Your Skin

OSPWs are vulnerable to sun damage, making daily sunscreen use an absolute necessity. However, since nearly all sunscreens contain oil, they can make your skin look shiny and cause your foundation and other makeup to streak. In addition, certain sunscreen ingredients can irritate your skin, leading to acne flare-ups. A list that follows of sunscreen ingredients to avoid is only for people who have sensitivity to sunscreens. If sunscreen sensitivity is not a problem for you, then there is no need to avoid these ingredients.

I recommend using physical blocking sunscreens that contain micronized zinc oxide and titanium dioxide. If you have darker skin, look for tinted products so you do not get the violet hue associated with the white cream products. And rather than creams, look for gel or foam sunscreens.

While I don't recommend tanning, much less burning, I know many of you are sun worshippers, and if you do wind up with a sunburn, take an Advil (ibuprofen) or aspirin every four hours to decrease inflammation and prevent redness. Using an over-the-counter 1 percent hydrocortisone cream may help heal sunburn as well.

### RECOMMENDED SUN PROTECTION PRODUCTS

- $ Aveeno Positively Radiant SPF 15 or 30 Moisturizer
- $ Blue Lizard Australian Suncream, SPF 30+, Sensitive
- $ Neutrogena Ultra Sheer Dry-Touch Sunblock Lotion SPF 85
- $ Purpose Dual Treatment Moisture Lotion SPF 15 UVA / UVB Sunscreen
- $ Alpha Hydrox Sheer Silk Moisturizer SPF 15 UVA/UVB Sunscreen & AHA
- $$ Minus-Sol Facial Sun Protection SPF 30+
- $$ Quintessence Sunshade SPF 30
- $$$ Caudalie Vinoperfect Day Perfecting Cream SPF 15
- $$$ Nia24 Sun Damage Prevention 100% Mineral Sunscreen
- $$$ SkinCeuticals Sheer Physical UV Defense SPF 50

**Baumann's Choice:** My patients with oily skin tell me they prefer Minus-Sol Facial Sun Protection SPF 30+.

**SUNSCREEN INGREDIENTS TO AVOID**

*If you have sunscreen sensitivity:*

- Avobenzone
- Benzophenones (such as oxybenzone)
- Methoxycinnamate (often found in waterproof sunscreens, can cause a reaction)
- Para-aminobenzoic acid (PABA)

If your skin is very oily, you can protect it while decreasing shine by mixing an equal portion of an oil control product in with your sunscreen and applying them together.

## Your Makeup

Powders containing sunscreen are made for OSPWs since they cover dark spots, control shine, and protect skin from the sun. If you use foundation to cover dark spots, look for an oil-free product with some of the anti-inflammatory ingredients I recommend.

### RECOMMENDED POWDER/ FOUNDATIONS AND FOUNDATIONS

- $  Organic Wear Pressed Powder
- $  Maybelline Pure Stay Powder & Foundation SPF 15
- $  Neutrogena SkinClearing Oil-Free or Foundation
- $  Neutrogena Healthy Skin Enhancer SPF 20
- $$  VMV Hypoallergenics Skin Savvy 60 Ultra-High Protection, Creamy Perfection, Liquid-Créme Foundation SPF 60
- $$  Bare Escentuals RareMinerals Skin Revival Treatment
- $$$  DiorSkin AirFlash Spray Foundation

**Baumann's Choice:** Neutrogena SkinClearing Oil-Free Pressed Powder has salicylic acid to help improve acne or skin redness.

## PROCEDURES FOR YOUR SKIN TYPE

If desired, you can augment the efficacy of your regimen with some simple cosmetic procedures. Due to the wrinkling to which this type is prone, OSPWs may wish to consider going for Botox or Dysport (botulinum toxins) and dermal fillers.

### Light Treatments

Intense Pulsed Light (IPL) can be used by your dermatologist to erase blood vessels and brown spots on the skin with minimal downtime. I happen to use the Cool Touch IPL by Cutera in my practice, but there are other types available. In addition, there are other devices utilizing blue light or red light, which can be used alone or with a photosensitizing agent called Levulan to treat acne and brown spots, and to shrink the size of the oil glands. For information on light treatments consult your dermatologist.

### Chemical Peels

In addition to the over-the-counter cleansers containing salicylic acid that I've recommended, OSPWs can also benefit from chemical peels performed in the dermatologist's office. These peels contain higher concentrations of salicylic acid (approximately 20–30 percent) than those found in consumer products (typically 0.5–2 percent). Peels are helpful for unclogging pores, clearing acne, and improving brown spots.

Light-skinned OSPWs will also benefit from deeper peels, such as the TCA or Obagi Blue Peel, which act on both dark spots and wrinkles. Costing between $200 and $400 per peel, they can be done every six months, and depending on the severity of the spots and wrinkles, you may need anywhere from two to four treatments.

Another option is facial masks performed at a salon or spa. Choose masks that are antioxidant, depigmenting, skin lightening, anti-inflammatory, or oil-decreasing.

Dark-skinned OSPWs can also benefit from *superficial* skin peels, such as those performed at salons or spas, while some of the deeper chemical peels are not right for dark-toned skin.

# Microdermabrasion

Instead of deep peels and light treatments, OSPWs with darker skin can use microdermabrasion, a process that blows aluminum, clay, or other types of particles against the skin to "sandblast" it. By taking off your skin's dead surface, microdermabrasion speeds up natural exfoliation, allowing the dead pigment-containing skin cells to flake off, so that brown spots disappear. Used in conjunction with retinoids, microdermabrasion may help the retinoid penetrate further, increasing its effectiveness in removing brown spots. You will benefit from microdermabrasion or light chemical peels with salicylic acid in concert with the regimen for combating dark spots.

Many salons and spas offer a series of ten weekly treatments at a cost of about $120 per session. Currently, at-home microdermabrasion kits have become available. These permit you to receive a similar benefit at a much lower cost.

## Ongoing Care for Your Skin

Changing your habits can do a lot to slow down the slippery slope that leads to premature aging. First, come in from the sun. Next, use the Daily Skin Care Regimen I've designed for you. Because of your skin's tendency to wrinkle, I highly recommend that you move up to prescription retinoid products sooner rather than later, as they will make a big difference. And finally, OSPWs can really benefit from the best that cosmetic dermatology has to offer. If you can afford it, consider what advanced procedures like Botox and wrinkle fillers can offer.

# CHAPTER FIVE

# Oily, Sensitive, Pigmented, and Tight: OSPT

## BAUMANN SKIN TYPE NUMBER 5

■

*"My oily skin troubles me. I know that sunscreen and skin light-*
*eners will help the dark patches on my skin, but it is so hard to find*
*products that do not make my face shiny or irritated. Please help!"*

### ABOUT YOUR SKIN

If you have an OSPT Skin Type, your skin's unique characteristics combine
to create a vicious cycle of blemishes, followed by brown spots, followed by
blemishes. Some people get acne and others get dark spots. OSPTs get
both. You may feel overwhelmed because you are always battling one kind
of outbreak or another. Nor will simple solutions aimed at one of your
skin's problems resolve the situation. You need to understand and address
all of them.

Pigmentation, sensitivity, and oil production are your skin's three dominant features. In this chapter, I'll first reveal how each factor affects your
skin, and then I'll show you how they interact. Yours is a complex type in
which your skin cycles through one form of skin reaction after another. But
don't worry, you can intervene and take charge of your skin.

### ONE PROBLEM AT A TIME

Let's begin with oil, your biggest concern. Your skin's oiliness can lead to
acne, especially during your adolescence and early twenties, with breakouts

continuing well into your thirties, and sometimes beyond. Although many people expect acne to end with youth, for OSPTs, it doesn't!

You may also find that your skin's pigmentation produces dark spots and melasma, dark patches on the skin. They too are worse in your twenties and thirties. Why? Because at that age, more women become pregnant or take birth control pills, or do both in turn, leading to hormone fluctuations, which stimulate oil production and pigmentation. Certain birth control pills will help acne by decreasing oil secretion, but can make more color and worsen melasma, due to their hormonal effects. Light-skin-toned OSPTs can often tolerate them, but those with darker skin tones may get undesirable pigmentation. In any event, the increased symptoms caused by hormonal levels will pass with time.

Address your challenges, or they can worsen. If you have acne, rosacea, or skin allergies, treatment is a necessity. You can decrease the reactive combination of oiliness, sensitivity, and pigmentation by following the protocols I'll offer later in this chapter. If you act to prevent breakouts and brown spots, you'll find that you can successfully manage your skin. Fortunately, many female OSPTs find that their skin improves after menopause, when oil production and hormones naturally level off.

By the time you get to your fifties and sixties, if you have protected your skin, your skin's good qualities will come to the fore. The oil production that has been your bane in youth becomes a balm as you age, preserving your skin's hydration. From midlife on, with minimal wrinkles, decreased oiliness, and reduced tendency to form dark spots, you enjoy skin that resists aging better than many other types. As others reach for the wrinkle creams (or other more advanced antiaging procedures), you will mature into the benefits that oily, tight skin confers over time.

## PIGMENT AWAY

Your second major challenge is pigmentation. Higher pigment levels can lead to unsightly dark spots that spring up suddenly and don't fade for weeks or even months. Pigment-producing cells in the skin can produce several different kinds of dark spots, which I detailed more fully in the section on pigmentation in Chapter Two.

Depending on your skin color and ethnic origin, you will get certain forms of pigmentation, but not others. Therefore, throughout this chapter, I'll discuss the best treatment options for the different types of pigmentation.

Dark spots of all types can develop from a wide range of factors, including inflammation, wounds, nicks, and cuts, as well as increased estrogen levels. In addition, sun exposure accelerates your skin's tendency to produce the pigment that creates dark spots, melasma, sun spots, and freckles.

## SPECIAL CHALLENGES OF YOUR SKIN TYPE

First, your skin's innate oiliness leads to a pimple, which is one form of inflammation. Next, the inflammation increases pigmentation at the site of the breakout, producing an unsightly dark spot in the exact location of the breakout.

This pattern of successive skin problems is frustrating. Whether your problem is acne, cuts, rashes, or allergic reactions, you breathe a sigh of relief that you've finally cleared it up, only to notice that you now must contend with dark spots. You may notice that these spots look worse and last longer than the original problem! Dermatologists call this condition post-inflammatory pigmentation alteration (PIPA). Fearing these spots will become permanent, people often refer to them as "scars." But your dark spots are not permanent, nor are they scars. By preventing inflammation, you can intervene in the vicious cycle, once and for all.

This sequence of skin problems can also appear anywhere on the body. People come to my office complaining they feel too embarrassed to wear skirts because a cut on their leg has turned into an unsightly dark area. This is a common experience for many OSPTs.

## OSPTs AND INFLAMMATION

Added to the above factors, the third element in your skin care challenge is your skin's sensitivity, which makes you more susceptible to inflammatory reactions that lead to dark spots. That's why it's essential to identify and avoid inflammatory triggers, so I'll identify a range of them for you here.

Inflammation is caused by the increased presence of red or white blood cells that rush to the site of an injury to aid in recovery. Pimples, burns, insect bites, bruises, rashes, and allergic reactions are common ones, but any type of inflammation, even blood cells concentrated at the site of a cut, can trigger the formation of brown spots. Any heat source outside the body can also increase inflammation *inside* the body.

External heat contributes to inflammation, which is why burns, hot wax applications, sunburns, and irritating skin care ingredients that cause redness can all lead to the OSPT vicious cycle. Sunning and burning on a hot day can also result in inflammation. Although skin pigmentation will prevent sunburns in dark-skinned OSPTs, the *heat* from sun can still be a problem.

Avoid sun exposure, hot weather, burns, and excess heat from all sources. Elective services, including waxing, saunas, steam rooms, peels, or other treatments that heat or irritate the skin can all provoke the inflammation cycle. So can these common cosmetic treatments:

- Plucking facial hair with tweezers can traumatize skin.
- Chemical depilatories that remove hair, like Nair, often contain strong chemicals that can irritate your skin.
- Hot waxes can create inflammation.
- Strong chemical peels are too harsh.
- Razors that promise a close shave increase the risk of developing ingrown hairs, which lead to inflammation.
- Hot, spicy food, drinks, and climate can cause inflammation.
- Saunas, body wraps, and hair treatments involving heat or harsh chemicals such as coloring, perming, or straightening can cause a problem.

## SKIN SENSITIVITY AND OSPTs

As a sensitive type, you're also more likely to develop redness, burning, stinging, rashes, or allergies in response to some skin care ingredients. Most people, including many skin service professionals, don't have a clue about which ingredients cause allergies or inflammations, so it's up to you to protect your skin from products and procedures that do more harm than good. Even products labeled hypoallergenic may contain fragrances or preservatives to which sensitive types react. Read the fine print and steer away from ingredients that might provoke a reaction. Later in this chapter, I will alert you to sensitizing ingredients and steer you toward skin care products and ingredients that will help calm, rather than provoke, inflammation.

In addition to the risk of product reactions, you may suffer from enhanced sensitivity to reactive agents from other sources. Although the topic is outside the scope of this book, it's not uncommon for allergic individuals to react to certain foods, fabrics, or chemicals present in clothing, furnishings, or buildings. For example, Karen, an attractive woman with freckles and green eyes inherited from her German grandmother, had also inherited Grammy's allergy to strawberries. When Karen ate them, she developed a small rash that disappeared within a few hours. Another type might have tolerated this passing reaction in order to enjoy a favorite fruit, but as an OSPT, Karen didn't have that luxury because the allergic reaction triggered an inflammatory–brown spot cycle. Some allergies are not as obvious as Karen's immediate reaction to strawberries, but can trigger a response hours or days later. If allergic reactions persist in expressing via your skin, consider working with a specialist in allergies to identify your triggers and avoid them.

## A CLOSE-UP LOOK AT YOUR SKIN

The OSPT Skin Type is quite common among people with medium and darker skin color, like Caribbean Americans, Latin Americans, Asians, and Mediterraneans. Lighter-skinned people from other ethnic backgrounds, like the Irish or English, can be OSPTs, as can a redhead with freckles, which are a form of pigmentation. If the questionnaire revealed that you're an OSPT, but you don't experience all the symptoms I'll cover, your test result isn't wrong. OSPTs share many common problems, but there are some differences, so throughout this chapter, I'll discuss the various symptoms, tendencies, and treatment options typical for dark-, medium-, and light-toned OSPTs.

All OSPTs are likely to experience:

- Acne, rashes, skin allergies
- Dark spots or patches in areas of sun exposure
- Shininess from sunscreen use
- Stinging or irritation from many skin care products

With dark-toned OSPT skin, you may also experience:

- Dark spots in areas of previous acne, irritation, or trauma (such as cuts, nicks, scrapes, and burns)
- Sunscreen appears white or purple when applied to skin
- Difficulty finding a facial foundation in the right shade in a product that your sensitive skin can tolerate
- Makeup used to cover dark spots causes oiliness, shine, or acne
- Ingrown hairs with resulting dark spots
- Dark circles under the eyes

Medium-toned OSPTs of Italian, Indian, Latin American, Asian, or other ethnicity may also experience:

- Oiliness, shine, or acne caused by makeup used to cover dark spots
- Dark circles under the eyes

Light-skinned OSPTs may also experience:

- Facial freckles
- Sun spots on hands, arms, and legs
- Increased risk for melanoma skin cancer, especially if you have red hair or freckles

Finding the right treatments is easier for light-skin-toned OSPTs whose freckles and sun spots are easily improved by sun avoidance and sunscreen use in combination with skin care treatments that I'll discuss in this chapter. Skin-bleaching agents are helpful for all OSPTs, but those with light skin tones can also use stronger treatments, such as lasers and light treatments. However, I never recommend those treatments for darker skin tones as they can lead back to that same vicious cycle of inflammation. If you are Asian, beware. Although your skin color may appear light, your skin may react to inflammation just like people with a darker skin tone. Follow the treatment recommendations for the dark- or medium-skin-toned OSPT groups.

Light-skinned OSPTs are at increased risk for melanoma skin cancers, especially if you have freckles and a history of sunburns. It's important to check moles yourself and also to have regular checkups by a dermatologist.

## SIGNS OF MELANOMA: THE A, B, C, AND D

- Asymmetry: One side of the mole is not a mirror image of the other side.
- Borders: The borders are not distinct. It is hard to tell where the mole starts and stops.
- Color: The presence of more than one color or black, white, red, and yellow hues
- Diameter: Larger than a quarter-inch

There is no way to prevent melanoma, although you can reduce your risk by avoiding sun exposure. Your best chance is to catch it early while it's curable. If you notice a suspicious mole, immediately see a dermatologist. It may save your life. Waiting even one day can make a difference.

## RECOMMENDATIONS FOR OSPT SKIN

You can prevent acne, redness, and rashes by using my recommended products, which walk the tightrope between avoiding potentially reactive ingredients and providing helpful oil-reducing and anti-inflammatory benefits. Second, sun exposure increases pigmentation, making regular sunscreen use essential. Third, manage stress and avoid all activities and skin care interventions that provoke inflammation. Taking the steps discussed below can make all the difference. Luckily for you, most of your type's key issues *are* preventable.

**Dr. Baumann's Bottom Line:** Prevention is key! Lessen skin irritation and the pigmentation that follows it by using a consistent anti-inflammatory prevention strategy.

## EVERYDAY CARE FOR YOUR SKIN TYPE

Depending on where you are in the inflammation–breakout–dark spot cycle, choose the appropriate treatment application.

Skin lightening and oil treatment products can help manage a wide range of typical OSPT symptoms, most of which are caused by pigmentation and overactive oil production. Depending on whether your skin is more oily or combination, you can use or omit optional products like toners and moisturizers.

If after using this regimen for six weeks to two months, you find you need further help, please make an appointment with a dermatologist. If your symptoms are acute, schedule an appointment at once, as there's often a waiting list.

I've provided different Daily Skin Care Regimens to address the different kinds of problems OSPTs experience. Select the right one, and then refer to the specific product recommendations that can be used with it.

Make it your daily habit to use the products that prevent your key problems. To this basic program, you can add supplementary treatment options when you have the specific problem they address.

## DAILY SKIN CARE

---

### REGIMEN FOR ACNE AND DARK SPOTS WITHOUT REDNESS:

| AM | PM |
|---|---|
| Step 1: Wash with cleanser | Step 1: Wash with cleanser |
| Step 2: Apply a toner (optional) | Step 2: Apply a toner (optional) |
| Step 3: Apply a skin lightener when you have dark spots (optional) | Step 3: Apply pimple medication when you have pimples (optional) |
| Step 4: Apply a benzoyl peroxide product to acne-prone areas | Step 4: If needed, apply a skin lightener to dark spots (optional) |
| Step 5: Apply an eye cream (optional) | Step 5: Apply an eye cream (optional) |
| Step 6: Apply sunscreen (non-optional!) | Step 6: Apply a moisturizer to dry areas if you have combination skin (optional) |
| Step 7: Apply SPF-containing makeup | |

---

In the morning, clean your face with a cleanser containing either salicylic acid or benzoyl peroxide. Complete facial cleansing with a toning product if your skin feels oily. (If your skin is less oily, you can omit this step.) If dark spots are present, apply a skin-lightening gel to them. If you are prone to acne or when you have active breakouts, apply a benzoyl peroxide–containing gel directly to the pimples. You can also use an on-the-spot pimple treatment product, which can be applied periodically during the day. Use an eye cream if you'd like to.

Next, apply your obligatory sunscreen and makeup, if desired.

In the evening, follow the same regimen, omitting the benzoyl peroxide gel and sunscreen and adding an eye cream and moisturizer if needed. To determine if moisturizers are right for you, please read the advice and product recommendations in the product sections following these regimens.

## REGIMEN FOR SKIN REDNESS AND DARK SPOTS WITHOUT ACNE:

| AM | PM |
|---|---|
| Step 1: Wash with cleanser | Step 1: Wash with cleanser |
| Step 2: Apply a toner (optional) | Step 2: Apply a toner (optional) |
| Step 3: Apply a skin lightener when you have dark spots (optional) | Step 3: If needed, apply a skin lightener to dark spots (optional) |
| Step 4: Apply an eye cream (optional) | Step 4: Apply an eye cream (optional) |
| Step 5: Apply sunscreen (non-optional!) | Step 5: Apply a moisturizer to dry areas if you have combination skin (optional) |
| Step 6: Apply SPF-containing makeup | |

In the morning, cleanse your face with a cleanser that contains ingredients right for your condition. For facial redness, use an anti-inflammatory cleanser. For dark spots, use a soy or niacinamide cleanser. If your skin has a high O/D score (34 or greater), follow with a toner. If dark spots are present, apply a skin-lightening gel to them. Apply eye cream, if you wish to.

Next, apply sunscreen. If your O/D score is less than 34, use a moisturizer or makeup foundation with sunscreen. If your O/D score is greater than 34, skip the moisturizer and use a sunscreen alone or makeup powder that contains sunscreen.

In the evening, follow the same regimen, omitting sunscreen and makeup, again including an eye cream and moisturizer if needed.

## REGIMEN FOR SKIN REDNESS AND DARK SPOTS WITH ACNE:

| AM | PM |
|---|---|
| Step 1: Wash with cleanser | Step 1: Wash with cleanser |
| Step 2: Apply a skin lightener when you have dark spots (optional) | Step 2: If needed, apply pimple medication to pimples (optional) |
| Step 3: Apply a pimple spot treatment to pimples (optional) | Step 3: If needed, apply skin lightener to dark spots (optional) |
| Step 4: Apply sunscreen (non-optional!) | Step 4: Apply a moisturizer to dry areas if you have combination skin (optional) |
| Step 5: Apply SPF-containing makeup | |

In the morning, use a salicylic acid cleanser or anti-inflammatory cleanser to clean your face. If dark spots are present, apply a skin-lightening gel to them. If you are having acne or active breakouts, apply a pimple-control product to pimples, and take it with you to use if needed during the day. Next, apply sunscreen and makeup if desired.

In the evening, follow the same regimen, omitting the sunscreen, and including a moisturizer if needed.

## Cleansers

Choose a nonirritating cleanser to remove makeup without stripping your skin's natural oils. This helps decrease or control skin sensitivity. If your cleanser is drying your skin, use it every other day, alternating with a cleanser designed for sensitive skin, like Olay Total Effects Anti-Aging Anti-Blemish Cleanser. Avoid cold creams and cream cleansers, which are too heavy for your oily skin.

Here I provide several different categories of cleansers: Choose a cleanser from the category that matches your chosen Daily Skin Care Regimen.

## RECOMMENDED SALICYLIC ACID–
## CONTAINING CLEANSERS

- $ Aveeno Clear Complexion Foaming Cleanser
- $ Black Opal Skin Perfecting Blemish Wash
- $ Clean & Clear Advantage Acne Cleanser
- $ Burt's Bees Natural Acne Solutions Purifying Gel Cleanser
- $ Neutrogena Oil-Free Acne Wash
- $ Olay Total Effects Anti-Aging Anti-Blemish Cleanser
- $$ Topix Gly/Sal 5-2 Cleanser

**Baumann's Choice:** Neutrogena Oil-Free Acne Wash

## RECOMMENDED BENZOYL PEROXIDE–
## CONTAINING CLEANSERS

- $ Clean & Clear Continuous Control Acne Cleanser
- $ Oxy Acne Treatment, Maximum Strength
- $$ PanOxyl Bar 5% (by Stiefel Laboratories)
- $$ Proactiv Renewing Cleanser

**Baumann's Choice:** PanOxyl Bar 5%

## RECOMMENDED CLEANSERS
## WITH SOY OR NIACINAMIDE

- $ Aveeno Positively Radiant Cleanser
- $ Olay Daily Facials Lathering Cloths for Sensitive Skin
- $ Neutrogena Visibly Even Foaming Cleanser

**Baumann's Choice:** Aveeno Positively Radiant Cleanser or Neutrogena Visibly Even Foaming Cleanser

## RECOMMENDED ANTI-
## INFLAMMATORY CLEANSERS

- $ Aveeno Ultra-Calming Foaming Cleanser
- $ Eucerin Gentle Hydrating Cleanser
- $ Topix Citrix Antioxidant Cleanser
- $$ Korres Pomegranate Cleansing and DeMake Up Wipes

**Baumann's Choice:** Korres Pomegranate Cleansing and DeMake Up Wipes because oily types who need to wash several times a day can use it on the go

## Toner Use

Oily types typically enjoy the clean and refreshing feeling that toners can provide. Also, anti-inflammatory, pigment, and oil-control substances in toners remain on the skin to deliver ingredients. However, if you have combination skin, avoid using toner on dry areas. If you experience redness or stinging when using skin care products such as moisturizers or sunscreens, omit toners and use a facial gel with anti-inflammatory ingredients. If your daily regimen gets too complicated, omit toner use.

### RECOMMENDED TONERS

$ Iman Perfect Response Gentle Toner for Acne Prone Very Oily Skin
$$ Paula's Choice Healthy Skin Refreshing Toner
$$ Arbonne NutriMin C RE$^9$ Restoring Mist Balancing Toner
$$ Josie Maran Argan Bear Naked Wipes
$$$ Erno Laszlo Conditioning Preparation Toner for Oily to Extremely Oily Skin

**Baumann's Choice:** Visitors to www.skintypesolutions.com with OSPT skin types chose Josie Maran Argan Bear Naked Wipes as their favorite toner. Come to the site and share your favorite.

## Handling Breakouts

Oily, sensitive types are vulnerable to breakouts, which may leave scars, especially if you pick at them or squeeze them incorrectly. The products in your daily regimen should help prevent them, and you can treat breakouts with some of the products listed on the following page, and then allow your body's natural healing process to resolve them.

Above all, don't steam your face, apply a hot washcloth, or place an ice cube on a pimple. All of these actions cause rapid changes in temperature, which is strictly a no-no for types prone to inflammation. Some believe that sun exposure will help clear up acne, but since acne typically worsens in summer, I don't believe that it's helpful.

The best thing to do is to leave a pimple alone and apply a pimple medication that contains salicylic acid or benzoyl peroxide.

### RECOMMENDED ACNE TREATMENT KITS

$ Clean & Clear Advantage 2-in-1 Acne & Mark Eraser Kit
$ Neutrogena Advanced Solutions Complete Acne Therapy System
$$ Rodan & Fields Unblemish Regimen
$$$ Triabeauty Be Clear Starter Kit

### RECOMMENDED ACNE CONTROL PRODUCTS WITH BENZOYL PEROXIDE

$ Oxy Vanishing 100% Fragrance Free Spot Treatment, Sensitive
$ Walgreens Maximum Strength Acne Medication
$ Zapzyt Acne Treatment Gel 10% Benzoyl Peroxide
$ PanOxyl Aqua Gel Benzoyl Peroxide 10%
$$ Jan Marini Benzoyl Peroxide 5%
$$ MD Formulations Benzoyl Peroxide 10%
$$ Proactiv Repairing Lotion

**Baumann's Choice:** No favorite, they're all good

### RECOMMENDED SPOT TREATMENTS FOR PIMPLES

$ Clean & Clear Clear Advantage Acne Spot Treatment
$ Burt's Bees Acne Spot Treatment
$ Neutrogena On-the-Spot Acne Treatment, Vanishing Formula
$ Biore Deep Cleansing Pore Strips Nose
$ Neutrogena SkinClearing Blemish Concealer
$$ La Roche-Posay Effaclar Al, Acne Treatment
$$ Exuviance Blemish Treatment Gel
$$$ Acne Solutions Anti-Blemish Post Blemish Formula
$$$ Guerlain Issima Crème Camphréa

**Baumann's Choice:** Neutrogena SkinClearing Blemish Concealer because it has salicylic acid. It not only conceals the blemish, but treats it as well.

# Treating Dark Spots

For dark spots, apply skin lightening products, making sure to use them after cleansing and toning but before other recommended products. Begin to use these products at the very first sign of darkening, and continue use until the spot has completely disappeared. You can also use them on dark spots you've had for some time.

### RECOMMENDED SKIN-LIGHTENING GELS

- $    Specific Beauty Skin Brightening Serum
- $    Skineffects by Dr. Jeffrey Dover Advanced Brightening Complex
- $$   Murad Age Spot & Pigment Lightening Gel
- $$   Paula's Choice Resist Remarkable Skin Lightening Lotion with 7% AHA
- $$   Peter Thomas Roth Radiance Oxygenating Serum
- $$$  DDF Fade Gel 4
- $$   Neostrada HQ Skin Lightening Gel
- $$$  Dr. Brandt Lightening Gel
- $$$  Dr. Michelle Copeland Age Spot and Pigment Lightening Formula
- $$$  Vivite Vibrance Therapy
- $$$  Purlisse Pur Bright Ultra Skin Brightening Serum

**Baumann's Choice:** Allergan (the Botox company) made another winner with Vivite Vibrance Therapy. It is expensive but this is an example of when it is worth it to splurge.


# Moisturizers

Unnecessary or disadvantageous for most OSPTs, moisturizers can clog your pores and increase oiliness. In most cases, your own naturally occurring oil is all you need. However, if you have some dry areas, around the eyes, cheeks, or jaw (or an O/D score between 27 and 35), apply a light moisturizing product with ingredients that work against inflammation, acne, and dark spots to the dry areas only or, if needed, to the entire face.

### RECOMMENDED MOISTURIZERS

- $    Aveeno Positively Radiant Anti-Wrinkle Cream
- $    Black Opal Advanced Dual Phase Fade Creme with Sunscreen

- $ Eucerin Redness Relief Daily Perfecting Lotion
- $ Avalon Organics CoQ 10 Wrinkle Defense Serum
- $ Yes to Cucumbers Facial Hydrating Lotion
- $$ Skyn Iceland Antidote Quenching Daily Lotion

**Baumann's Choice:** Yes to Cucumbers Facial Hydrating Lotion was a favorite with OSPT skin types who follow us on www.facebook.com/BaumannCosmetic.

## Eye Creams

For dark circles under your eyes, use eye creams containing vitamin K, which may address the blood congestion that is thought to cause them.

### RECOMMENDED EYE CREAMS

- $ RoC Retinol Correxion Eye Cream
- $$ Nia24 Eye Repair Complex
- $$ Skineffects by Dr. Jeffrey Dover Eye Effects Dual Action Under Eye Therapy
- $$ Elizabeth Arden Ceramide Eyewish SPF 10
- $$$ Canyon Ranch Your Transformation Brightness Eye Cream
- $$$ Murad Lighten and Brighten Eye Treatment

**Baumann's Choice:** Murad Lighten and Brighten Eye Treatment works in four to six weeks to lighten dark circles. You must take a one-month holiday from this every three to four weeks to keep it working well.

## Exfoliation

Using a facial scrub helps certain types, but it's not beneficial for OSPTs because vigorous exfoliation can lead to inflammation and dark spots. If you use retinoids, you'll find that they naturally exfoliate the skin.

## SHOPPING FOR PRODUCTS

Widen your choice of products by reading labels to determine product ingredients, so that you can select those that contain beneficial ingredients while avoiding ones that increase inflammation or oiliness. If you find products that you like that are not listed here; please visit www.skintypesolutions.com and tell me your favorites so I can pass them along to others of your Skin Type. Check the ingredients in your shampoos, conditioners, bubble baths, and shaving products as well, as these contact your skin and can cause irritation.

## SKIN CARE INGREDIENTS TO USE

### To decrease skin inflammation:

- Aloe vera
- *Arctium lappa* (burdock root)
- *Boswellia serrata*
- Chamomile
- Cucumber
- Dexpanthenol (pro-vitamin $B_5$)
- *Glycyrrhiza glabra* (licorice extract)
- Licochalone
- Mallow
- Niacinamide
- Red algae
- Rose water
- Salicylic acid (beta hydroxy acid, or BHA)
- Silymarin
- Sulfacetamide
- Sulfur
- Tea tree oil
- Zinc

### To lessen acne:

- Azelaic acid
- Benzoyl peroxide (unless you experience facial redness)
- Resorcinol (dark-skinned OSPTs should use with caution)
- Retinol
- Salicylic acid (beta hydroxy acid, or BHA)
- Tea tree oil (can cause allergy in some people)

### To prevent pigment:

- Niacinamide

### To reduce pigment:

Use when you have dark spots, melasma, or undesirable pigmentation

- Arbutin
- Azelaic acid
- Kojic acid
- Mulberry extract

- Bearberry extract
- Cucumber extract
- *Epilobium angustifolium* (willow herb)
- *Glycyrrhiza glabra* (licorice extract)
- Resorcinol (dark-skinned OSPTs should use with caution)
- Salicylic acid (beta hydroxy acid, or BHA)

## SKIN CARE INGREDIENTS TO AVOID

### Cleansing Ingredients to Avoid

- Avoid any products that have thick, "vigorous" foam.

### If acne prone:

- Butyl stearate
- Cinnamon oil
- Cocoa butter
- *Cocos nucifera* (coconut oil)
- Decyl oleate
- Isocetyl stearate
- Isopropyl isostearate
- Isopropyl myristate
- Isopropyl palmitate
- Isostearyl isostearate
- Isostearyl neopentanoate
- Jojoba oil
- Myristyl myristate
- Myristyl propionate
- Octyl palmitate
- Octyl stearate
- Peppermint oil

### If you have skin allergies or rashes:

- Benzoyl peroxide
- Fragrances
- Lanolin
- Parabens
- Propylene glycol-2 (PPG-2)

## Sun Protection for Your Skin

Often light-skinned OSPTs avoid the sun because they know that they will just burn and freckle. Thanks to the unique combination of oiliness and pigmentation, OSPTs with medium skin tone can achieve a glowing, gorgeous tan. However, medium- and dark-toned OSPTs should wear sunscreen to prevent the formation of dark spots, which are caused by UVB and UVA light. That's why a broad-spectrum sunscreen, which blocks both UVA and UVB rays at all times, is a must, regardless of your skin color. Because OSPTs have oily skin, gels, light lotions, and sprays will feel better than greasy creams and lotions. OSPT skin is sensitive, so physical barrier sunscreens that contain titanium dioxide and zinc oxide are better than chemical sunscreens that can sting and burn. You will notice you may still get a light tan, as no sunscreen blocks 100 percent of the sun's rays.

And remember, if you have an outbreak of melasma or acute sun spots, total sun avoidance is best. For extra "security," choose a product that offers anti-inflammatory and skin lightening ingredients as well as sun protection.

## RECOMMENDED SUN PROTECTION PRODUCTS

$ Aveeno Positively Radiant Daily Moisturizer SPF 15 (with UVA-UVB protection)
$ Neutrogena Healthy Defense Liquid Moisturizer SPF 50
$ Olay Total Effects 7x Visible Anti-Aging Vitamin Complex with UV Protection
$$ Minus-Sol Ivory Facial Sun Protection SPF 30+

**Baumann's Choice:** Aveeno Positively Radiant Daily Moisturizer SPF 15 or 30 because it contains Total Soy Complex, which helps prevent dark patches from forming

### SUNSCREEN INGREDIENTS TO AVOID

Due to skin sensitivity, some OSPTs experience stinging, burning, and redness in reaction to certain ingredients commonly used in sunscreens. If this occurs, stop using the offending product immediately and avoid these ingredients:

• Avobenzone
• Benzophenone
• Butyl methoxydibenzoyl methane
• Isopropyldibenzoylmethane
• Methylbenzylidene camphor
• Octyl methoxycinnamate
• Para-amniobenzoic acid (PABA)
• Phenylbenzimidazole sulfonic acid

## Your Makeup

You can cover a pimple, dark spots, or redness with makeup that contains certain key ingredients that prevent these same problems. For acne control, look for products that contain salicylic acid (such as Neutrogena Skin-Clearing Oil-Free Makeup), which improves acne, increases skin exfoliation, and decreases oiliness. To prevent dark spots, look for foundations with sunscreen. Although you need more sun protection than a foundation can supply, every bit helps. Most cosmetic lines contain three different foundation lines: one with oil, one without, and one with some added value, such as sunscreen. The oil-free version is best for you. Bypassing foundation altogether and instead using a powder with sunscreen is another good option.

OSPTs with darker skin tones will need to find foundation brands with a range of darker shades. Iman Cosmetics (found at Walgreens and Target) specializes in foundations for darker skin tones, so choose an oil-free product that matches yours.

Facial powders can temper your skin's shininess, if the recommended lotions and gels do not fully prevent it. As an added benefit, facial products that contain sunscreen will shield your skin from rays that stimulate pigmentation.

### RECOMMENDED FACIAL POWDERS WITH SUNSCREEN

$  Maybelline Pure Stay Powder SPF 15
$$  Avene Tinted Compact SPF 50
$$  tarte provocateur SPF 8
$$  Estée Lauder Double Wear Stay-in-Place Powder Makeup SPF 10
$$  Jane Iredale's Amazing Base Loose Minerals SPF 20

**Baumann's Choice:** Any are fine but do not rely on the sun protection in these powders.

### RECOMMENDED FACIAL POWDERS WITH ACNE OR OIL CONTROL

$  Avon Mark Matte-nificent Oil-Absorbing Powder
$  Maybelline Shine Free Oil Control Loose Powder
$  Neutrogena SkinClearing Pressed Powder

$$ Bobbi Brown Sheer Finish Loose Powder
$$ Jane Iredale Pure Matte Finish Powder
$$ Sephora Brand Mineral Double Compact Foundation SPF 10
$$ Stila sheer pressed powder
$$$ Lancôme Dual Finish Fragrance Free Powder
$$$ Shu Uemura Face Powder Matte

**Baumann's Choice:** Jane Iredale Pure Matte Finish Powder because it is specially formulated for those with acne

### RECOMMENDED FOUNDATIONS

$ CoverGirl Clean Oil-Control Makeup (for light coverage)
$ Iman Second To None Oil-Free Makeup, SPF 8 (for darker-skinned people)
$ Neutrogena SkinClearing Oil-Free Compact Foundation (for acne)
$ Revlon Colorstay for Combo/Oily Skin Makeup with SoftFlex SPF 6
$$ Dermablend Smooth Indulgence Foundation
$$ i.d. bareMinerals Foundation—SPF 15
$$ M·A·C Studio Fix
$$ Make-up Forever Mat Velvet + Matifying Foundation
$$ Clinique Acne Solutions Liquid Makeup
$$$ Chantecaille Real Skin Foundation

**Baumann's Choice:** Clinique Acne Solutions Liquid Makeup

## PROCEDURES FOR YOUR SKIN TYPE

In most cases, OSPTs with dark skin get the best results with topical products, while most medical procedures are unnecessary, and sometimes harmful. However, you'll need patience because topicals require time to effect a change.

In general, dark-skin-toned OSPTs should avoid light therapy because it can lead to inflammation and worsening of dark spots. The sole exception is blue light therapy, which kills bacteria and helps with acne. Typically, you would go once to twice per week for six weeks. The cost is approximately $150 per treatment and it may be covered by your insurance.

On the other hand, if your skin tone is light to medium-light (ranging in skin tones from someone like Nicole Kidman on the light end to someone like Jennifer Lopez at the medium-light end) you have the option of Intense Pulsed Light treatments (IPL) performed by a dermatologist. Lighter-skinned OSPTs are less prone to inflammation than dark-skinned OSPTs and can benefit from IPL and other forms of light therapy to lighten dark spots more rapidly, in addition to blue light treatments for acne.

## Additional Options

People with darker skin tones, or those who do not want (or cannot afford) IPL, can benefit from chemical peels. Look for ones that contain salicylic acid (BHA) of 20 percent or 30 percent, which removes the top layers of the skin and triggers the cells to divide faster, thereby encouraging brown spots to depart through the natural process of cell renewal. Resorcinol can also effectively treat acne and dark spots in OSPTs. If you have darker skin, make certain that you go to a dermatologist who is skilled at treating people with darker skin, because dark spots can worsen if chemical peels are not done correctly. These peels range from $120 to $250 per peel and you will typically require a series of five to eight sessions.

## ONGOING CARE FOR YOUR SKIN

Preventing the breakout–inflammation–brown spot cycle is the best strategy for OSPTs. To do that, follow the Daily Skin Care Regimen I've devised for you, and use my product recommendations. If you'd like, try a few simple procedures as well. Above all, make sure to avoid inflammation, eat the right foods, and de-stress whenever you can. By developing the right habits in youth, you can solve your skin problems. Managing this Skin Type definitely requires some effort, but over time, you'll come to appreciate your skin. In your later years, unlike some other Skin Types, you'll bypass costly antiaging routines and look good throughout life.

# CHAPTER SIX

# Oily, Sensitive, Non-Pigmented, and Wrinkled: OSNW

## BAUMANN SKIN TYPE NUMBER 8

■

*"My face often has redness or acne. It is embarrassing . . . and I am unsure which antiaging products to use that will not irritate my sensitive skin."*

### ABOUT YOUR SKIN

When the late English playwright Noël Coward wrote his famed and devastatingly witty song "Mad Dogs and Englishmen (Go Out in the Midday Sun)," he undoubtedly had OSNWs in mind. The intrepid English with their insistence on sunning at noon, are indeed a nation of OSNWs, as are many people from Scottish, Irish, German, and Scandinavian backgrounds. Fair skinned, with little pigment to handle sun exposure, what they lack in melanin, they make up for in dogged determination—they will produce a suntan where none is possible. This Skin Type also suffers from flushing and rosacea, but wrinkling most commonly results from sun damage.

### DON'T TAN, DON'T BURN

When they wrote the Coppertone ad jingle "Tan, Don't Burn," they weren't talking about your type. You *always* burn in response to moderate to maximum sun exposure. The many OSNWs I see in my practice come to me with wrinkles, redness, and rosacea resulting from a bad mix of genetic predisposition and harmful behavior. For you, sun avoidance is an absolute must.

Why?

As Coward mentions in the lyrics of his song, centuries of genetic adaptation did not prepare even pigmented types (like the Asians, Indians, and Hispanics to whom Coward refers in his lyrics) for the tropical sun. That's why they wisely stay indoors during the heat of the day. Meanwhile, the foolhardy Brits (and other melanin-deprived OSNWs) are determined to brave it, to their detriment.

With less pigmentation to protect you, the results are disastrous. Although I don't recommend tanning for anyone, when pigmented types tan, at least they have a chance to work *with* the sun, by starting with short sun exposure at times of the day when the rays are less harmful (such as before ten AM and after four PM). Then, as their pigment is activated, it provides some protection as they gradually increase exposure.

But most OSNWs lack both the genes to tan and the common sense as to how to go about it. After spending a year at a deskbound job, OSNWs will rush out to the beach, like lemmings to the sea, thinking to make up for the time spent indoors in one big blast. Instead, the pale, unprotected, unpigmented skin of the OSNW burns to a bright red. One or more burns over a lifetime will predispose skin to both non-melanoma skin cancers and the wrinkles that plague this type.

Some tan believing that sun is "good for the skin" or improves acne. Not true. UV radiation was shown to cause changes in the skin's natural oils that led to an *increased* number of blackheads. And studies also report a higher incidence of acne in the summer months.

## THE R-WORD, ROSACEA

Another prime reason to make sunscreen use a daily habit is that sun exposure causes breakage in blood vessels that can result in rosacea symptoms, such as flushing and facial redness. This occurs because sun exposure accelerates collagen loss, weakening the supportive structures around the blood vessels. In fact, a growing body of medical evidence indicates that in many instances rosacea is *caused* by sun damage.

OSNW skin is one of the types most prone to rosacea. If you've consulted a dermatologist, you may have received that diagnosis. Research shows that although fourteen million Americans suffer from rosacea, 78 percent of Americans are not aware of the disease—and many who have it do not realize that they do.

# What Is Rosacea?

The four common symptoms of rosacea are:

1. Facial redness and flushing
2. Acne with pimples and papules
3. Visible facial blood vessels
4. Enlarged oil glands that cause the nose to redden and thicken

You can have one or more of these symptoms simultaneously, and each symptom requires a different treatment. But having one symptom does not necessarily mean that you will develop the others. If you experience any of these rosacea symptoms, seek help sooner rather than later because receiving treatment can prevent rosacea from developing to its later stages.

The later stages of the disease can and should be avoided. One of the most well-known rosacea sufferers was the comedian W. C. Fields. The bulbous nose that contributed to his comic appearance is actually a telltale rosacea symptom, one that can be treated, if necessary, but is best prevented. The treatments I'll offer in this chapter will help do that.

## A CLOSE-UP LOOK AT YOUR SKIN

It's stressful to have rosacea. Studies indicate that rosacea sufferers commonly experience low self-esteem. When rosacea acts up, people want to hide. But if you have it, it's better to face facts and get treatment.

Although not every OSNW has rosacea, if you are on the rosacea spectrum with any of the common OSNW symptoms, my treatment protocols will help.

If you have OSNW skin and rosacea, you may experience any of the following:

- Facial redness and flushing
- Pink patches
- Difficulty tanning, frequent sunburns
- Pimples
- Facial oiliness
- Enlarged pores
- Facial rashes or pink scaling patches, especially around your nose
- Visible red or blue facial blood vessels

- Acne, burning, redness, or stinging in response to many skin care products
- Yellow or skin-colored bumps with a dent in the middle (These enlarged oil glands are called sebaceous hyperplasia.)
- Enlarged nose
- Wrinkles, frown lines, and crow's-feet
- Increased risk of non-melanoma skin cancer (basal cell carcinoma and squamous cell carcinoma)

Most OSNWs experience redness and flushing. "My face looks red in photos" is a common complaint. You may also notice yellowish bumps on your face with central indentations. These are enlarged oil-producing glands that over time may cause your nose to appear enlarged. Sun exposure worsens rosacea and all the symptoms on the rosacea spectrum.

## YOUR SKIN CARE HISTORY

Most OSNWs who come to my office have seen several dermatologists before finding their way to me, often suffering from decades of skin problems. Before the age of thirty, acne is an OSNW's biggest skin issue. Long considered a teenager's condition that passes with time, many people find it endures. The thirties can be tough because that's when the sebaceous glands are at their largest, making even more oily sebum. Experimenting with products may make matters worse, because sensitive skin reacts to many skin care ingredients.

OSNWs over forty may still suffer from acne or rosacea. Plus, in your thirties and forties (and, alas, sometimes even your twenties), wrinkles begin to appear as well. It can seem like the worst of all possible worlds. One positive note is that the oiliness causing acne tends to decrease in women in their forties and fifties due to menopause. (Sorry, men, your oil glands do not slow down until you are in your eighties.)

**Dr. Baumann's Bottom Line:** Following your Daily Skin Care Regimens and strict sun avoidance will help prevent your worst skin problems. Don't experiment with antiaging products. Follow my recommendations, find what works for you, and stop wasting money on expensive skin care products. Instead the right procedures will make the biggest difference.

## EVERYDAY CARE FOR YOUR SKIN

Your primary concerns are oiliness and facial redness, along with the tendency to develop broken blood vessels on your face. You therefore need nonirritating/anti-inflammatory products that will limit acne and redness. To find them, you may have tried products marketed for "sensitive skin," but found them irritating or overly oily since many sensitive skin products are better suited for those with dry skin.

Whether you have active rosacea, acne, or simply experience facial redness, breakouts, facial stinging, or rashes, the two regimens described in this section of the chapter will benefit you, and should be used on a daily basis.

Please look over the two regimens I provide. After you've determined which one is right for your needs, you can follow the same basic instructions for either regimen.

If after using either or both of these regimens for six weeks to two months, you find you need further help, consult a dermatologist, who can offer prescription cleansers, oral medications, and procedures that may make a huge difference for your Skin Type. If your symptoms are acute, you may wish to schedule an appointment at once, as there is often a waiting list.

## DAILY SKIN CARE

### REGIMEN FOR FLUSHED SKIN:

| AM | PM |
|---|---|
| Step 1: Wash with anti-inflammatory cleanser | Step 1: Wash with anti-inflammatory cleanser |
| Step 2: Apply antiaging serum | Step 2: Apply serum or moisturizer |
| Step 3: Apply moisturizer (optional) | Step 3: Apply retinol product |
| Step 4: Apply facial foundation with SPF or a gel sunscreen | |

## REGIMEN FOR ACNE:

### AM

Step 1: Wash with benzoyl peroxide cleanser

Step 2: Apply spot treatment to pimples

Step 3: Apply antiaging serum

Step 4: Apply moisturizer (optional)

Step 5: Apply facial foundation with SPF product or a gel sunscreen

### PM

Step 1: Wash with benzoyl peroxide cleanser

Step 2: Apply serum or moisturizer with anti-inflammatory ingredients

Step 3: Apply retinol product

Used morning and evening, a cleanser with anti-inflammatory ingredients and/or benzoyl peroxide will address acne by cutting down on skin surface oil. Those containing salicylic acid are also a good option. If you have only slightly oily skin you may choose to apply a moisturizer. If so, choose one with anti-inflammatory ingredients. If you have a higher O/D score (35 or above) and shiny skin, skip this step.

In the evening, use a cleanser to gently remove makeup. Then apply a light nighttime serum or a mask, lotion, or gel with anti-inflammatory ingredients. To help prevent wrinkles, use an anti-aging serum in the morning and a retinol product at night.

## Cleansing

I do not recommend toners for your type because they can increase flushing, so never use them. If you have a medium S/R score (25–33) and acne is your main problem, you can use scrubs, but no more than two to three times a week. Make sure to apply gently to avoid provoking inflammation. I am not a big fan of scrubs for your Skin Type, but some of you can use them if you follow these precautions. Do not use scrubs if your S/R score is higher than 33, or if you have redness and rosacea. You can use foaming cleansers, selecting one targeted to your main problem. For example, if you have acne, choose an acne wash, or if you have rosacea, look for cleansers that improve redness, such as Aveeno Ultra-Calming Foaming Cleanser.

## RECOMMENDED CLEANSING PRODUCTS

$   Aveeno Ultra-Calming Foaming Cleanser
$   Bioré Revitalize 4-in-1 Self Foaming Cleanser
$   Eucerin Redness Relief Soothing Cleanser
$   Say Yes to Cucumbers Calming Facial Cleansing Gel
$   Neutrogena Healthy Skin Anti-Wrinkle Anti-Blemish Cleanser
$   PCA Skin pHaze 31 BPO 5% Cleanser
$$   Citrix Antioxidant Cleanser
$$   Clarins Gentle Foaming Cleanser Combination/Oily Skin
$$   Topix Benzoyl Peroxide 5% Wash
$$   Lancôme Clarifiance Oil-Free Gel Cleanser
$$   Peter Thomas Roth Beta Hydroxy Acid 2% Acne Wash
$$   B. Kamins Booster Blue Rosacea Cleanser
$$$   Freeze 24/7 Skin Glace Daily Detoxifying Cleanser and Mask

**Baumann's Choice:** Freeze 24/7 Skin Glace Daily Detoxifying Cleanser and Mask

## RECOMMENDED SCRUBS

$   Avon Clearskin Professional Deep Pore Cleansing Scrub
$   Bioré Pore Perfect Pore Unclogging Scrub
$   Clean & Clear Blackhead Clearing Scrub
$   Burt's Bees Citrus Facial Scrub
$   Neutrogena Oil-Free Acne Wash, Redness Soothing Gentle Scrub
$   Skin Effects by Jeffrey Dover Purifying Effects Deep-Cleansing Enzyme Scrub
$$   Anthony Logistics for Men Facial Scrub
$$   Vivite Exfoliating Facial Cleanser

**Baumann's Choice:** Vivite Exfoliating Facial Cleanser is good if you have acne. If you have redness or rosacea, avoid scrubs.

## Acne Control Products

You can use these products when you have active acne, but I don't recommend squeezing pimples.

## RECOMMENDED ACNE TREATMENTS

- $ Neutrogena Oil-Free Acne Wash
- $ PanOxyl Bar 5% by Stiefel
- $ Paula's Choice 2% Beta Hydroxy Acid Liquid
- $$ Avon Clearskin Overnight Blemish Treatment
- $$ Exuviance Blemish Treatment Gel
- $$ Rodan & Fields Unblemish Dual Intensive Acne Treatment
- $$$ Erno Laszlo Total Blemish Treatment

**Baumann's Choice:** PanOxyl Bar 5% with benzoyl peroxide

## RECOMMENDED PIMPLE CONCEALER/TREATMENTS

- $ Almay Clear Complexion Concealer w/ Salicylic Acid
- $$ Neutrogena SkinClearing Blemish Concealer w/ Salicylic Acid
- $$ Clinique Acne Solutions Concealing Stick
- $$ Dr. Brandt Pores No More Pore Refiner
- $$$ Jurlique Blemish Cream

**Baumann's Choice:** Almay Clear Complexion Concealer w/ Salicylic Acid

## Moisturizers

Moisturizers are unnecessary for most oily types. However, wrinkles and redness, prime concerns for OSNWs, are often addressed via moisturizers, so I'll make some recommendations while warning you away from products that could worsen your sensitive skin. If your skin is very oily (with an O/D score over 34), look for serums, fluids, or lotions.

Products with anti-inflammatory ingredients can be used both to treat active redness and to calm your skin to prevent flushing and skin sensitivity. Once redness calms, you can prevent wrinkles with the antioxidant moisturizers and serums.

To prevent wrinkles, many OSNWs experiment with antiaging products, but these may contain harsh ingredients, like fruit acids and other active ingredients, that can irritate OSNW skin, causing acne, facial burning, or redness.

Instead use moisturizers and serums with antioxidants, which have been shown to prevent wrinkles and other signs of aging. In addition, I recommend that you increase antioxidant foods and even take an antioxidant supplement.

Since you will not be using toner, serums (and if desired, certain moisturizers) are an ideal delivery system for OSNW skin because they often contain a higher percentage of the active ingredients that penetrate better to combat wrinkles. But beware of ingredients that cause inflammation. The trick is to combine the right cocktail of ingredients, including those strong enough to work tempered by others that soothe irritation.

Powerful and costly antioxidants, like green tea, are more concentrated in serums and also stay on your skin longer than when used in cleansers, which rinse off. Delivered via a dropper-style bottle, serums are thick in texture, so that a little goes a long way. Use only a few drops and spread over your face.

Looking ahead, some moisturizers currently being developed will contain higher amounts of active ingredients; however, these may be pricey. While antioxidants help prevent wrinkles, those of you over thirty may choose retinol and prescription retinoids to help get rid of wrinkles that you already have.

## RECOMMENDED ANTI-INFLAMMATION MOISTURIZERS

- $ Aveeno Ultra-Calming Moisturizing Cream
- $ Eucerin Redness Relief Soothing Night Creme
- $$ Green Tea Botanicals Green Tea Anti-Aging Moisturizer SPF 30
- $$ Clinique CX Soothing Moisturizer
- $$ La Roche-Posay Rosaliac Skin Perfecting Anti-Redness Moisturizer
- $$ Paula's Choice HydraLight Moisture•InfusingLotion Normal to Oily/Combination Skin
- $$$ REN Hydra-Calm Global Protection Day Cream (not for acne)

**Baumann's Choice:** Aveeno Ultra-Calming Moisturizing Cream, which contains the herb feverfew, with antioxidant and anti-inflammatory properties

## RECOMMENDED SERUMS AND MOISTURIZERS

- $ Aveeno Ultra-Calming Moisturizing Cream with SPF 15
- $ Olay Regenerist Fragrance-Free Regenerating Serum
- $$ Benev Azalex Gel
- $$ iS Clinical Hydra-Cool Serum
- $$ Kirkland Signature By Borghese Advanced Age-defying Wrinkle Defense Serum
- $$ Caudalíe Face Lifting Serum with Grapevine Resveratrol

$$ Clarins Skin Beauty Repair Concentrate
$$ Elizabeth Arden Ceramide Advanced Time Capsules
$$ Pevonia Botanica RS2 Concentrate
$$ Murad Sensitive Skin Soothing Serum
$$ Tolerance Extreme Cleansing Lotion by Avene
$$$ Combray by Solenne
$$$ Jurlique Herbal Recovery Gel
$$$ SkinCeuticals Serum 10

**Baumann's Choice:** Olay Regenerist Daily Regenerating Serum because the niacinamide treats inflammation and may help prevent skin cancer

### RECOMMENDED WRINKLE TREATMENT PRODUCTS

$$ Afirm 3x (contains retinol)
$$ La Roche-Posay BioMedic Retinol 30
$$ Philosophy Help Me (contains retinol)
$$ Replenix Retinol Smoothing Serum 2x or 5x

**Baumann's Choice:** All products containing retinol are good when packaged in small-mouthed aluminum tubes that minimize air exposure.

## Eye Creams

Eye creams are not always necessary. I personally choose to use a regular facial moisturizer around my eyes. However, if you prefer a separate eye cream you can look for these products and use them before your moisturizer.

### RECOMMENDED EYE CREAMS

$ Derma E Pycnogenol Eye Gel with Green Tea Extract
$ Clinique All About Eyes Serum De-Puffing Eye Massage
$$ CosMedix Opti Crystal Eye Serum
$$ Jo Malone Green Tea and Honey Eye Cream
$$ Laura Mercier Eyedration
$$ Osmotics Blue Copper 5 Firming Eye Repair
$$ Obagi Elastiderm Eye Treatment Cream

**Baumann's Choice:** Obagi Eliastiderm Eye Treatment Cream because several of my patients have raved about it

## Masks

Use masks when you're flared with acne or redness, or otherwise about once or twice a week.

### RECOMMENDED MASKS

- $   Paula's Choice Skin Balancing Carbon Mask
- $$   Kiehl's Soothing Gel Masque
- $$   Peter Thomas Roth Therapeutic Sulfur Masque Acne Treatment
- $$   Proactive Refining Mask
- $$$   Laura Mercier Hydra Soothing Gel Mask

**Baumann's Choice:** Peter Thomas Roth Therapeutic Sulfur Masque because the sulfur helps decrease redness

## SHOPPING FOR SKIN CARE

You can widen your choice of products by reading labels to determine product ingredients, so that you can select those that contain beneficial ingredients for you, while avoiding ones that may cause irritation, inflammation, or oiliness. If you find products that you like that are not on my lists, please go to www.skintypesolutions.com and share your finds with other OSNWs.

---

### SKIN CARE INGREDIENTS TO LOOK FOR

*Antioxidants to prevent wrinkles:*

- Basil
- Caffeine
- *Camilla sinensis* (green tea, white tea)
- Coenzyme $Q_{10}$ (ubiquinone)
- Grape seed extract
- Idebenone
- Lutein
- Lycopene
- Pomegranate

- Feverfew
- Genistein
- Ginger
- Ginseng
- Pycnogenol (a pine bark extract)
- Silymarin
- Yucca

### To decrease inflammation:

- Aloe vera
- *Arctium lappa* (burdock root)
- Basil
- *Boswellia serrata*
- Chamomile
- Dexpanthenol (also known as provitamin B$_5$)
- *Epilobium angustfolium* (willow herb)
- Feverfew
- Ginger
- Licochalone
- Mallow
- Niacinamide
- Red algae
- Salicylic acid (beta hydroxy acid, or BHA)
- Sulfacetamide
- Sulfur
- Tea tree oil
- Zinc

### To improve acne:

- Benzoyl peroxide (but see below)
- Retinol
- Salicylic acid (beta hydroxy acid, or BHA)
- Tea tree oil

### COMMON BEAUTY PRODUCT NO-NO'S

- Acetone
- Alcohol
- Benzoyl peroxide (see below)

## A No-No for Many OSNWs: Benzoyl Peroxide

Benzoyl peroxide (BP) is one of the most commonly used topical preparations for acne. It helps fight bacteria and moderates oiliness. Although it works, it may cause burning, stinging, and redness in sensitive OSNW skin. However, not all OSNWs will experience this problem, and many individuals who suffer from acne will benefit from its use. People with lower

S/R scores (from 30 to 34) may be able to use benzoyl peroxide. Also it may be easier to tolerate a product like Proactiv Repairing Lotion because it contains a lower concentration of BP (2.5 percent or less). Combining a benzoyl peroxide product with an anti-inflammatory product such as Cutanix Sensitive Skin Moisturizer may help you use benzoyl peroxide.

## SKIN CARE INGREDIENTS TO AVOID

### *Due to stinging and itching from skin care products:*

- Acetic acid
- Balsam of Peru
- Benzoic acid
- Cinnamic acid
- Lactic acid
- Menthol
- Parabens
- Quaternium-15

### *To minimize pimples or blackheads:*

- Butyl stearate
- Chemical additives such as decyl oleate, isocetyl stearate, isopropyl myristate, isostearyl neopentanoate, isopropyl isostearate, isopropyl palmitate, myristyl myristate, myristyl propionate, octyl palmitate, octyl stearate,
- and propylene glycol-2 (PPG-2)
- Cinnamon oil
- Cocoa butter
- *Cocos nucifera* (coconut oil)
- Lanolin
- Peppermint oil

### *To minimize skin redness:*

- Alpha hydroxy acids (lactic acid, glycolic acid)
- Alpha lipoic acid
- Benzoyl peroxide (for some people)
- Vitamin C

## Sun Protection for Your Skin

Tanning is not for you. But so many forces in our society drive women to want to look like models, actresses, or people they see on television. I believe in being yourself, and using the best of skin care to enhance who you are.

You need to wear sunscreen at all times except at night. Use an SPF of

15 daily, and when outside, or in a sunny climate, use an SPF of 45–60. Smooth a quarter-size portion of product over the entire face, neck, and chest every morning. If you are in the sun for longer than one hour, reapply sunscreen every hour. To get the most benefit from sunscreens apply them after cleansing to reduce surface skin oiliness. Lotion or gel sunscreens are better choices for you than cream sunscreens, because creams will make your skin look oilier. Powders that contain sunscreen are also a great option.

## RECOMMENDED SUN PROTECTION PRODUCTS

- $  Aveeno Ultra-Calming Daily Moisturizer with SPF 15
- $  Eucerin Sensitive Facial Skin Extra Protective Moisture Lotion with SPF 30
- $  RoC Age Diminishing Daily Moisturizer SPF 15
- $$  Kiehl's Ultra Protection Water-Based Sunscreen SPF 25
- $$  Philosophy Supernatural, Poreless, Flawless SPF 15
- $$  La Roche-Posay Anthelios 60 Ultra Light Sunscreen Fluid for Face
- $$$  Lancôme Bienfait Multi-Vital SPF 30
- $$  iS Clinical SPF 25 Treatment Sunscreen

**Baumann's Choice:** Aveeno Ultra-Calming Daily Moisturizer with SPF 15 because it contains the herb feverfew, which has both antioxidant and anti-inflammatory actions

### SUNSCREEN INGREDIENTS TO AVOID

*If skin burns, itches, or turns red
in response to sunscreen, avoid:*

- Avobenzone
- Benzophenone
- Octyl methoxycinnamate

## Your Makeup

Since talc helps control oil, pressed powder, powdered eyeshadow, and blush will absorb oil and last longer. According to the National Rosacea Foundation, mineral makeup can help people with rosacea since it's nonirritating and naturally protective to the skin. Although some companies claim that their makeup offers sun protection as well, I recommend applying mineral makeup over your sunscreen to assure that you have the right degree of sun protection.

### RECOMMENDED MAKEUP FOUNDATIONS

- $ Ideal Shade Cream-to-Powder Foundation SPF 15
- $$ Revlon Colorstay for Combo/Oily Skin Makeup with SoftFlex SPF 6
- $$ Neutrogena SkinClearing Oil-Free Makeup
- $$ Philosophy The Supernatural Airbrushed Canvas Powder Foundation

**Baumann's Choice:** Philosophy The Supernatural Airbrushed Canvas Powder Foundation has an SPF of 15 and absorbs oil well.

### RECOMMENDED POWDERS

- $ L'Oréal Idéal Balance Pressed Powder for Combination Skin with SPF 10 Sunscreen
- $ Neutrogena SkinClearing Mineral Powder
- $$ Revlon ColorStay Pressed Powder
- $$ Illuminants Brilliant Finish SPF 25 Powder Foundation

**Baumann's Choice:** Revlon ColorStay Pressed Powder. Increase your sun protection by dusting an SPF-containing powder over your sunscreen. This will help prevent shine from the sunscreen and give you some added protection.

### RECOMMENDED FACIAL POWDERS WITH SUNSCREEN

- $ Maybelline Pure Stay Powder SPF 15
- $ Neutrogena Mineral Sheers Loose Powder Foundation SPF 20
- $$ Illuminants Brilliant Finish SPF 25 Powder Foundation
- $$ Jane Iredale's Amazing Base Loose Minerals SPF 20

**Baumann's Choice:** They are all good. Jane Iredale's is available from your dermatologist.

---

**SKIN CARE INGREDIENTS TO AVOID**

*Foundation:*

- Oil

*Powder:*

- Avoid pressed powders with isopropyl myristate. Look for oil-control products instead.

*Blush:*

- Avoid D & C red dyes (xanthenes, monoazoanilines, fluorans, and indigoids).
- Look for the natural red pigment carmine instead.

---

## PROCEDURES FOR YOUR SKIN

As an OSNW, you have three main problems—facial redness, overactive oil glands, and wrinkles—and my procedure recommendations will help treat all three. In your type, after your blood vessels dilate, they do not constrict properly as they do in other types.

Intense Pulsed Light Treatments (IPL) may help decrease wrinkles long-term by stimulating fibroblasts, the skin cells in the dermis that make collagen. Short-term, IPL causes slight swelling that puffs out your fine wrinkles and smoothes your skin's texture. Although future research will evaluate whether this treatment has any long-term antiwrinkling effect, its benefits for the treatment of facial flushing and visible blood vessels are well established.

However, please note that the rosacea and aging process will most likely continue despite these treatments, necessitating future treatments and current prevention strategies. Although capable of thwarting the progression of aging and rosacea, the procedures I recommend will not end it permanently.

## IPL and Vascular Lasers

Another approach for flushing, redness, visible blood vessels, and other symptoms on the rosacea spectrum combines Intense Pulsed Light (IPL) with various vascular lasers. They work synergistically to reduce blood vessels and facial flushing symptomatic of rosacea.

## Treating Advanced Rosacea

Most of the recommended procedures also work for dilated blood vessels. They cost between $400 and $500, and are not usually covered by insurance. Although it may require two to five treatments for the vessels to disappear, once vessels disappear, they are usually gone permanently. An annual maintenance treatment can treat any new ones that appear.

There are several different options for treating the enlarged nose that may occur with more advanced rosacea, including surgery, dermabrasion, and $CO_2$ laser. Please consult with your dermatologist.

## Other Treatment Options

For more advanced options to remove wrinkles, you can consider cosmetic procedures, such as the use of Botox and dermal fillers. However, make sure that you have substantially reduced your rosacea and flushing first. As a precaution, be aware that you will be more likely than other types to experience redness due to the rubbing and the use of ice and anesthetic creams that occur during the procedures. However, the redness usually resolves in about twenty minutes.

## ONGOING CARE FOR YOUR SKIN

Coming in from the midday sun (or indeed, any sun) is absolutely critical for your sensitive, redness-prone skin. Wear sunscreen regularly, and adhere to your daily regimen to address your skin care problems. Anti-inflammatory and antioxidant foods and ingredients in skin care products can help tremendously. Don't experiment with antiaging products. The right procedures (Botox, dermal fillers, and Intense Pulsed Light) will help resolve your type's most persistent issues.

# CHAPTER SEVEN

# Oily, Sensitive, Non-Pigmented, and Tight: OSNT

## BAUMANN SKIN TYPE NUMBER 6

∎

*"My skin is oily and sensitive but luckily I do not have an issue with wrinkles yet. I need help finding products that will soothe my irritated skin. I am tired of wasting money on products that do not work."*

### ABOUT YOUR SKIN

As an OSNT, your biggest problem is facial flushing, which never fails to give you away in social situations. No one wants the world to know their secrets, but OSNTs are walking lie-detector tests, as their face reveals everything they feel.

Tense at the meeting? It shows on your face. Attracted to that new acquaintance? It's hard to hide. If you need a cool head or an impassive look, you'd better forget about it. Your face will always give you away, and you just have to learn to deal with it by relaxing, doing things you find calming, and avoiding ingredients, products, and (when possible) life situations that are inflammatory. Don't worry, it's not that you're thin-skinned. You may suffer from rosacea, a dermatological condition, common among OSNTs, that affects fourteen million Americans.

### THE R-WORD

OSNT skin is a perfect setup for rosacea, pronounced rose-AY-sha. Despite the scientific terminology, rosacea is really a collection of symptoms that you may know well. While approximately 78 percent of Americans have never heard of this condition, it's vital to recognize and treat it early to slow the disease process. By identifying which symptoms trouble you, you can manage them or, in some cases, eliminate them and thereby prevent later-stage symptoms.

How does flushing occur? First, blood vessels dilate more in sensitive types due to heightened sensitivity to neurotransmitters (similar to hormones). Second, like Bill Clinton, many OSNTs have light skin, which reveals the redness of dilated blood vessels more readily than dark skin. Over time, blood vessels lose their ability to contract back to their normal size, so they remain dilated. These visible red or blue blood vessels look like spider veins. Many people of Irish and Scottish descent have the OSNT type, as do members of my own family. To find out if you have rosacea, please consult Chapter Six, "The R-Word, Rosacea."

Doctors believe that certain symptoms can lead to others. For example, frequent facial flushing can lead to broken blood vessels, which many sufferers complain about often saying, "they make me look like an alcoholic." But don't worry; they can be eliminated using Intense Pulsed Light technology. I've treated literally thousands of people, both men and women, for this problem.

If you are an OSNT with darker-toned skin who experiences the same burning and stinging but without the visible flushing and dilated blood vessels, you'll find my daily regimens, product recommendations, and lifestyle guidelines helpful. The procedures for treating more intensive rosacea symptoms are not necessary.

If you're Asian and your test results indicated that you are an OSNT, you should double-check your answers because a special trait common to Asians could produce misleading scores. Many Asians lack an enzyme that processes alcohol, causing flushing when they drink. So if you're Asian and you flush only when you drink, you're probably not a true OSNT. Most Asians fall into the pigmented category, and worry more about dark spots than wrinkles.

If you have an S/R score of 34 or higher, you may experience one (or more) inflammatory skin problems: rosacea, acne, skin allergies, and burning in response to some skin care ingredients. Whatever the cause, my recommendations will help you.

If you have severe acne, excess hair on your face, and irregular menstrual periods, it could also indicate an underlying medical condition known as polycystic ovarian syndrome. If you've had trouble treating acne and suffer from these other symptoms, please consult a gynecologist.

## A CLOSE-UP LOOK AT YOUR SKIN

With OSNT skin, you may experience any of the following:

- Facial redness and flushing
- Pimples
- Facial oiliness
- Pink patches
- Yellow or skin-colored bumps with a dent in the middle (These enlarged oil glands are called sebaceous hyperplasia.)
- Acne, burning, redness, or stinging in response to many skin care products
- Facial rashes or pink scaling patches, especially around your nose
- Difficulty tanning, frequent sunburns
- Visible red or blue facial blood vessels

Although rosacea and rosacea-like symptoms can be uncomfortable and embarrassing, they occur within an overall pattern of skin oiliness and sensitivity that you can treat and prevent. Also, facial redness is not always due to rosacea. For example, it's not uncommon for sensitive types to react to harsh chemicals. Some people are allergic to the nickel in the little ball that helps mix the nail polish when you shake the bottle. The new euro coin also has a high nickel content, and when people with nickel allergies handle these coins and then touch their faces, redness and irritation can result.

All by themselves my daily regimens will help many OSNTs, but keep in mind that people with highly reactive skin often have specific allergies beyond those mentioned. If you follow my guidelines, and notice no change in your skin reactivity, you may want to consult an allergist to identify allergies to specific foods, products, or environmental factors.

## OSNTs AND AGING

Hormones regulate the production of your skin's oil, or sebum. In the human life cycle, birth is an initial high point in oil production, with a second taking place between the ages of nine and seventeen—the acne years. Thereafter, oil production normalizes at adult levels. In women, sebum levels begin to fall during menopause. In men, this decrease is deferred until their eighties. In other words, the oiliness of OSNT skin improves with time (and women improve sooner than men). As you age, the acne caused by overactive oil production usually lessens. Finally, a benefit to going through menopause! However, women aren't out of the woods, since the hot flashes that some women experience can result in increased facial flushing—your biggest complaint.

To prevent or reduce the signs of aging, many people use antiaging skin creams, but OSNTs should stay away from them. You don't need them, and their fruit acids and other ingredients can irritate your skin. Their exfoliation action is good for others, but not for you. Your best age prevention technique is the regular use of sunscreen and anti-inflammatories in your skin care and diet.

Believe it or not, the OSNT Skin Type is a great one to have. Younger OSNTs may not believe me, but all I can say is: Wait until you're forty.

When other types are scrambling to minimize the signs of aging, you'll look in the mirror with gratitude for your youthful looks. Believe me, a lot of people would trade places with you! One of the great assets of this type is that you rarely wrinkle. What's more, your skin is free of the dark spots and blotches that mar so many people's complexions.

OSNTs will save a fortune because aging will not bring the wrinkles and sags that drive others to costly procedures like Botox, collagen injections, face-lifts, and microdermabrasion. If you read other chapters of this book, you'll see that I don't hesitate to advise antiaging treatments when necessary. But I have a different message for OSNTs: Don't waste your time or money on those costly procedures. You don't need them. You can skip facials, facial steaming, chemical peels, and microdermabrasion. Are any advanced skin care options right for your Skin Type? Yes, and in the procedure section of this chapter, you'll find effective interventions for your main problems—redness, flushing, and acne.

## NON-MELANOMA CANCER

Light-skinned OSNTs with a history of excess sun exposure are at risk for non-melanoma skin cancer. Even though you're less likely to wrinkle or get dark spots, you should always wear sunscreen to prevent skin cancer.

## How to Recognize a Non-Melanoma Skin Cancer

There are two types of non-melanoma skin cancer, so make sure to check yourself for both kinds regularly.

1. Squamous cell carcinoma (SCC): SCC commonly appears as a red, scaling patch that scabs in sun-exposed areas, such as the face, ears, chest, arms, legs, and back. Although they resemble scabs, unlike scabs, they do not heal. An SCC may also be covered by a hard white scale that resembles a wart. Consult a dermatologist if you have a spot that fits this description and persists for three months or more.

2. Basal cell carcinoma (BCC): BCCs are bumps that look white, shiny, and luminous like a pearl. They usually appear with a central raised ridge. Another variation is tiny blood vessels which appear around their borders. BCCs may also resemble a crater that shows up suddenly and resembles a scar, though no trauma or injury has caused it. Sometimes the border is "ruffled," or heaped up around the central crater.

**Dr. Baumann's Bottom Line:** Save money on skin products, but never skimp on sunscreen.

## EVERYDAY CARE FOR YOUR SKIN

What skin care products best serve your needs? Your primary concerns are oiliness, facial redness, and inflammation, along with the tendency to develop broken blood vessels. You therefore need nonirritating products that will limit acne and redness. If you've tried products marketed for "sensitive skin," you may have found them irritating or overly oily since these products are usually formulated for dry skin.

I've provided three different regimens. If you experience facial redness, breakouts, facial stinging, rashes, or active rosacea, use the first one daily. Use the second regimen if you have active acne. Use the maintenance regimen when your problems have cleared. Next, you can choose the products you'll need from those I recommend in each category later in this chapter.

If after following these regimens for six weeks, you find you need further help, consult a dermatologist.

## DAILY SKIN CARE

### REGIMEN FOR ROSACEA AND REDNESS:

| AM | PM |
|---|---|
| Step 1: Wash with cleanser | Step 1: Wash with cleanser |
| Step 2: Apply an anti-inflammatory gel or lotion | Step 2: Apply an anti-inflammatory product |
| Step 3: Apply an oil control product (optional) | |
| Step 4: Apply sunscreen | |
| Step 5: Apply oil-free foundation or powder with sunscreen | |

In the morning, wash with cleanser and apply an anti-inflammatory gel or lotion. If you have a high O/D score (above 35), you can apply an oil-control product before putting on sunscreen and makeup. Always use a sunscreen, even if you spend the day indoors.

In the evening, cleanse to gently remove makeup. Then apply a light nighttime lotion or gel with anti-inflammatory ingredients. Use masks or peels when skin is flared with acne or redness, and lotions and gels for maintenance when skin is calm. If your skin is less oily (with an O/D score of 27–35), choose lotions over gels. OSNTs with a higher score (above 35) may prefer gels.

### REGIMEN FOR ACNE:

| AM | PM |
|---|---|
| Step 1: Wash with cleanser | Step 1: Wash with cleanser |
| Step 2: Apply spot treatment for pimples | Step 2: Apply anti-inflammatory gel |
| Step 3: Apply oil-control product | Step 3: Apply a retinol product |
| Step 4: Apply oil-free foundation or powder with sunscreen | Step 4: Apply moisturizer (optional if skin feels dry) |

In the morning, wash with cleanser and use spot treatment for pimples, if needed. Then apply an oil-control product before putting on sunscreen and makeup. Always use a sunscreen.

In the evening, use a cleanser to gently remove makeup. Then apply a light nighttime mask, lotion, or gel with anti-inflammatory ingredients. Use masks when skin is flared with acne or redness, or serums for maintenance when skin is calm. If you scored between 27 and 35, your skin is slightly more combination, and serums are a better choice, as the recommended masks may be too drying. OSNTs with higher O/D scores (above 35) can benefit from both serums and masks.

---

**REGIMEN FOR MAINTENANCE WHEN ACNE AND REDNESS ARE UNDER CONTROL:**

| AM | PM |
|---|---|
| Step 1: Wash with cleanser | Step 1: Wash with cleanser |
| Step 2: Apply oil-control product | Step 2: Apply anti-inflammatory gel |
| Step 3: Apply oil-free foundation or powder with sunscreen | Step 3: Apply a retinol product |
| | Step 4: If skin feels dry, apply moisturizer |

In the morning, wash with cleanser and apply an oil-control product before putting on sunscreen and makeup.

In the evening, use a cleanser to gently remove makeup. Then apply a light nighttime mask, lotion, or gel with anti-inflammatory ingredients. Wait three to five minutes, and then follow with a retinol-containing product. Next, you can use a moisturizer if your skin feels dry or if you scored between 27 and 35 on the O/D questions.

## Cleansers

My recommended cleansers contain anti-inflammatory ingredients that cut down on skin surface oil. Those with salicylic acid, sulfacetamide, or sulfur are a good option.

## RECOMMENDED CLEANSING PRODUCTS

- $   Cetaphil Daily Facial Cleanser, Normal to Oily Skin
- $   Eucerin Redness Relief Soothing Cleanser
- $   Neutrogena Oil-Free Acne Wash
- $   Olay Total Effects Anti-Aging Anti-Blemish Daily Cleanser
- $   PanOxyl Bar 5% by Stiefel
- $   Paula's Choice Hydralight One Step Face Cleanser Normal to Oily/Combination Skin
- $$   DDF Salicylic Wash 2%
- $$   Philosophy On a Clear Day Super Wash for Oily Skin
- $$   Murad Redness Therapy Soothing Gel Cleanser
- $$   Rodan & Fields Soothe Gentle Cream Wash
- $$   Vichy Normaderm Deep Cleansing Gel
- $$$   Pevonia RS2 Gentle Cleanser

**Baumann's Choice:** Paula's Choice Hydralight One Step Face Cleanser Normal to Oily/Combination Skin

## Toners

Most OSNTs won't need toners, which can worsen the flushing and redness you experience, because they often contain ingredients (like menthol) that can trigger flushing. People with severe rosacea should totally avoid toners.

However, if you like toners, choose ones with anti-inflammatory ingredients, like witch hazel. If cosmetic products often cause redness or stinging, a toner designed for sensitive skin such as Skin Medica Acne Treatment Toner is one option.

## Acne-Prone OSNTs

With acne but only minimal facial flushing and redness, you can use products containing benzoyl peroxide. The popular Proactiv system, composed of various benzoyl peroxide treatments, is geared toward this type. Any of their products can be substituted or combined with the other recommendations in this chapter. However, you can't buy the treatments individually; you must buy the entire kit, and it's not cheap. Many similar products containing benzoyl peroxide are available by prescription, which could save you money.

## RECOMMENDED ACNE PRODUCTS

$   Clean & Clear Advantage Acne Spot Treatment
$   Burt's Bees Natural Acne Solutions Targeted Spot Treatment
$   Neutrogena On-the-Spot Acne Treatment
$   PanOxyl Bar 5% by Stiefel
$$   Kinerase Clear Skin Blemish Dissolver
$$   DDF Benzoyl Peroxide Gel
$$   Kiehl's Blue Herbal Spot Treatment
$$   Peter Thomas Roth AHA/BHA Acne Clearing Gel
$$   Philosophy On a Clear Day Blemish Serum
$$$   Murad Exfoliating Blemish Gel
$$$   La Roche-Posay Effaclar Al, Acne Treatment

**Baumann's Choice:** DDF Benzoyl Peroxide Gel. However, this product may be too strong for very sensitive types. If you find it irritating, look for products with 2.5 percent benzoyl peroxide.

## Flushing- and Redness-Prone OSNTs

OSNTs with flushing and redness may not tolerate high-strength benzoyl peroxide products and the other acne treatments mentioned above. Instead, look for products with licochalone, feverfew, and other anti-inflammatory ingredients.

## RECOMMENDED ANTI-INFLAMMATORY PRODUCTS

$   Aveeno Ultra Calming Moisturizing Cream
$   Eucerin Redness Relief Soothing Night Creme
$   Paula's Choice Skin Relief Treatment
$$   Clinique CX Redness Relief Cream
$$   Josie Maran Argon Oil
$$   Origins Mega-Mushroom Skin Relief Advanced Face Serum

**Baumann's Choice:** Eucerin Redness Relief Soothing Night Creme because it contains licochalone, or Aveeno products with the anti-inflammatory herb feverfew

## Moisturizers

Due to your skin's naturally occurring oil, moisturizers may clog your pores and increase oiliness. However, if you have an O/D score of 27–35, you may use a light moisturizer that also contains ingredients that minimize inflammation and acne. But make sure to apply it to the dry areas only.

### RECOMMENDED MOISTURIZERS FOR REDNESS

- $  Aveeno Ultra-Calming Moisturizing Cream
- $  CeraVe Moisturizing Lotion
- $  Eucerin Redness Relief Daily Perfecting Lotion
- $$  Clinique CX Redness Relief Cream
- $$  Rosaliac Anti-Redness Moisturizer

**Baumann's Choice:** Rosaliac Anti-Redness Moisturizer by La Roche-Posay because it contains thermal water with selenium, both of which are good anti-inflammatory ingredients

### RECOMMENDED MOISTURIZERS FOR COMBINATION SKIN

- $  Aveeno Ultra-Calming Moisturizing Cream
- $  CeraVe Moisturizing Lotion PM
- $  Eucerin $Q_{10}$ Anti-Wrinkle Sensitive Facial Skin Creme
- $  Paula's Choice Skin Balancing Moisture Gel
- $$  Eminence Rosehip Whip Moisturizer
- $$  fresh Umbrian Clay Face Lotion
- $$$  Kate Somerville Oil Free Moisturizer

**Baumann's Choice:** CeraVe Moisturizing Lotion. They have a great night cream with niacinamide as well.

## Peels

Discuss with your dermatologist or aesthetician whether or not you should use peels. If recommended, ask for peels with anti-inflammatory ingredients such as sulfur and salicylic acid.

## Masks

Masks are helpful when your skin is especially oily. You can use a mask prior to an important event or even daily—there's no harm done with frequent application.

### RECOMMENDED MASK PRODUCTS

$ Burt's Bees Healthy Treatment Pore Refining Mask
$$ Astara Blue Flame Purification Mask
$$ DDF Sulfur Therapeutic Mask
$$ bliss Steep Clean Mask
$$ SkinCeuticals Clarifying Clay Masque

**Baumann's Choice:** DDF Sulfur Therapeutic Mask

## Skin Exfoliation

I recommend skin exfoliation only for certain types, and OSNTs should definitely avoid it because vigorous exfoliation can lead to inflammation. Always treat your skin as gently as possible, using only soft washcloths to wash your face. Avoid any harsh facial cleansing products, such as disposable facial cleansing cloths and cleansing pillows. These products are designed to be slightly abrasive and are not for you.

## SHOPPING FOR PRODUCTS

Your recommended skin care products contain anti-inflammatory ingredients to calm your skin's redness. Widen your selection by reading ingredient labels to include additional products with beneficial components. Always avoid products with ingredients that could cause irritation, inflammation, or oiliness. If you find products that you like that are not on my product lists, please go to www.skintypesolutions.com and tell me what treasures you have found.

## SKIN CARE INGREDIENTS TO USE

- Aloe vera
- Chamomile
- Cucumber
- Dexpanthenol (pro-vitamin B$_5$)
- Feverfew
- *Glycyrrhiza glabra* (licorice extract)
- Licochalone
- Niacinamide
- Salicylic acid (beta hydroxy acid, or BHA)
- Tea tree oil
- Zinc

## SKIN CARE INGREDIENTS TO AVOID

- Acetic acid
- Allantoin
- Alpha lipoic acid
- Balsam of Peru
- Benzoic acid
- Camphor
- Cinnamic acid
- Cinnamon oil
- Cocoa butter
- *Cocos nucifera* (coconut oil)
- DMAE
- Isopropyl isostearate
- Isopropyl myristate
- Lactic acid
- Menthol
- Parabens
- Peppermint oil
- Quaternium-15

## Sun Protection for Your Skin

To get the most benefit from sunscreens, apply after cleansing to reduce surface skin oiliness. Lotions or gels are better for you than cream sunscreens.

Apply additional sunscreen even if using an SPF makeup (foundation or powder). Smooth a quarter-size portion of product over your entire face, neck, and chest. Reapply after six hours or every hour if you are out in direct sun. For complete instructions on sunscreen use, please reread Chapter Two. Please note that the list on the following page of sunscreen ingredients to avoid is only for people who have sensitivity to sunscreens. Several sunscreens I recommend for this type contain certain of these ingredients, so if you do have sunscreen sensitivity—read the label before buying.

## RECOMMENDED SUN
## PROTECTION PRODUCTS

$  Aveeno Ultra-Calming Daily Moisturizer SPF 15

$  Eucerin Sensitive Facial Skin Extra Protective Moisture Lotion
with SPF 30

$  Blue Lizard Australian Suncream, SPF 30, Baby

$  Neutrogena Sensitive Skin Sunblock Lotion SPF 60+

$  Purpose Dual Treatment Moisture Lotion with SPF 15

$$  La Roche Posay Anthelios 60 Ultra Light Sunscreen Fluid

$$  Prescriptives All You Need + SPF 15 Continuous Action 24-Hour
Moisture for Oilier Skin

$$  VMV Hypoallergenics Armada Face and Body Shield 60

$$  SkinCeuticals Sheer Physical UV Defense SPF 50

**Baumann's Choice:** Whatever you choose, use it every day.

---

### SUNSCREEN INGREDIENTS TO AVOID

*If you have sunscreen sensitivity:*

- Avobenzone
- Benzophenone
- Butyl
  methoxydibenzoylmethane
- Isopropyl dibenzoylmethane
- Methylbenzylidene
  camphor

- Octyl methoxycinnamate
- Para-amenobenzoic acid
  (PABA)
- Phenylbenzimidazole
  sulfonic acid

---

## Your Makeup

OSNTs benefit from makeup with ingredients to minimize, treat, or conceal skin problems. Depending on which problems are paramount, you can select from various options.

For redness around the eye area, use an under-eye concealer with anti-inflammatory ingredients such as Neutrogena's Skin Soothing Eye Tints. People with a high O/D score (over 34) may prefer powders to foundations, while those with scores lower than 34 may like the coverage of a foundation. For acne or rosacea, look for foundations and powders with salicylic acid, such as Neutrogena SkinClearing Oil-Free powder and foundation.

In general, OSNTs benefit from using medicated facial powders, especially if you have acne. But if you need to cover flushing or blemishes, choose an oil-free, yellow-tinted foundation that helps mask the redness, such as Giorgio Armani Fluid Sheer Foundation #6 formula. Or else apply a tinted makeup primer, such as Biotherm's Pure Bright Moisturizing Makeup Base with a purple tint to cover redness. O/D scores over 34 may find this product too oily, but if you've scored in the 27–33 range, you may enjoy its coverage.

If eyelid redness is a problem, avoid shiny, frosted, or iridescent eye shadows. The rough edges of the ingredients used to give the product shimmer may cause skin irritation. Powder eye shadows and blushes are recommended rather than cream products, because creams may streak on oily skin.

## RECOMMENDED FOUNDATIONS

$ L'Oréal Infallible Advanced Never Fail Makeup SPF 20
$ Neutrogena SkinClearing Oil-Free Makeup
$$ Boots No7 Intelligent Balance Mousse Foundation
$$ M·A·C Studio Fix Powder Plus Foundation
$$$ Giorgio Armani Fluid Sheer

**Baumann's Choice:** Boots No7 Intelligent Balance Mousse Foundation. This is from the UK. Boots is available at Target. The entire Boots No7 line is great! Check www.skintypesolutions.com for updates.

## RECOMMENDED POWDERS

$ Almay Clear Complexion Pressed Powder
$ Neutrogena SkinClearing Oil-Free Pressed Powder
$$ VMV Hypoallergenics Oil-Absorbing, Clarifying, Pore-friendly Pressed Powder
$$ Laura Mercier Foundation Powder
$$$ Lancôme Ageless Minérale with White Sapphire Complex

**Baumann's Choice:** Almay Clear Complexion Pressed Powder

## PROCEDURES FOR YOUR SKIN TYPE

Sulfur, sulfacetamide, and antibiotic-containing skin care products as well as the oral medications, available through your dermatologist, can help treat the flushing and acne forms of rosacea. Blue or red light therapy can also help reduce acne. The light therapy works by killing facial bacteria that causes acne. You can schedule treatments every two weeks for a series of ten to twelve treatments.

At this time, no topical or oral product is available to successfully treat the two other symptoms of rosacea: the dilated blood vessels (spider veins) and the yellowish, enlarged nose with large pores. A number of dermatological office procedures are effective in treating the dilated blood vessels, including the electric needle, an injection of saline solution, a laser, or a light device such as Intense Pulsed Light (IPL).

Most of the recommended procedures for dilated blood vessels cost between $400 and $500. They are not usually covered by insurance, and it typically takes from two to five treatments for the vessels to disappear. But rest assured that these treatments are worth it, because once vessels disappear, they are gone permanently, and an annual maintenance treatment can handle any new ones that appear.

## IPL and Levulan

My preferred procedure for rosacea spectrum is using IPL and Levulan together. They work synergistically to reduce the oil, blood vessels, and yellow papules that are symptomatic of rosacea. Your skin's oil-producing glands and red blood vessels absorb Levulan, which makes them more sensitive to light. Then, when the IPL is flashed on the skin, it shrinks and partially destroys them. The end result is that oil glands are less able to produce oil. This helps to eliminate yellow papules, the enlarged oil glands that so many OSNTs complain about. In addition, the IPL erases many of the visible facial blood vessels and improves pink cheeks. This occurs because the enlarged blood vessels take up the heat of the light and it destroys them, leaving normal skin untouched.

## Treating Advanced Rosacea

There are several different options for treating the enlarged nose that may occur with more advanced rosacea. Please refer to page 102 for my suggestions.

## Cosmetic Procedures to Avoid

Although you may be tempted by a variety of services and products promising to help you address skin care problems, most of the following are a waste of time and money:

- Microdermabrasion is too harsh for your sensitive skin.
- Facials are too heating and inflammatory for your redness-prone skin.
- Non-ablative lasers, except those designed to improve rosacea and get rid of blood vessels, are more geared to wrinkles; you don't need them.

In addition, you probably do not need either Botox or fillers such as collagen and hyaluronic acid because you don't have wrinkles. However, they can be used to change eyebrow shape or make the lips bigger if desired.

## Ongoing Care for Your Skin

Since the OSNT Skin Type is on the rosacea spectrum, your skin will never be as trouble-free as other types. However, if you follow my program and treat problems early, in most cases, you will be able to avoid the more advanced stages of rosacea. I see many OSNTs (both men and women) since what I offer is the most effective approach. So feel confident in following my recommendations. And as I've mentioned, if you begin taking good care of your skin now, you have something you can look forward to. Your skin will improve with age.

## PART THREE

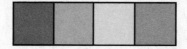

# Skin Care for Oily, Resistant Skin

# CHAPTER EIGHT

# Oily, Resistant, Pigmented, and Wrinkled: ORPW

## BAUMANN SKIN TYPE NUMBER 11

■

*"My skin is fairly easy but I need advice on how to have a more even complexion and prevent unwanted skin aging. Do these antiaging creams really work? I am not sure they do anything for my skin."*

## ABOUT YOUR SKIN

Put down that magnifying mirror! It will only reveal what you already know. If your questionnaire results showed that you have ORPW skin, it's no surprise that you have ongoing skin care challenges. There is hardly any skin issue from which you are exempt (except for skin sensitivity), and picking at your face will not solve the problem.

I can't guarantee that the oiliness, enlarged pores, and dark spots that have marred your complexion since adolescence can be cured in an instant, nor will your skin problems disappear with age. However, for ORPW women, skin oiliness *will* lessen in midlife, although it can leave enlarged pores and acne scars in its wake. What's more, the aging process will result in wrinkling. Yes, ORPWs, you get a hit on both sides of the youth-age spectrum.

## FREE TO EXPERIMENT

All ORPWs are at risk for wrinkles. But if you quit smoking and sunning, the right skin care products can help alleviate your skin problems. But be warned: Most over-the-counter products will not be sufficiently concentrated for your tough all-weather skin!

Resistant skin has one significant upside: It's nonreactive. That means you can experiment with different products without negative responses. For you, no rashes, no burning or stinging—all hallmarks of skin sensitivity. Sensitive types get paranoid about products, afraid to try new things. But you can freely sample different products at department store cosmetic counters. You can wash your face with any soap that's handy. When visiting relatives or staying in a hotel, you can use the shampoo without experiencing dryness or irritation.

Your Skin Type proves why "one size fits all" skin care can never work. While sensitive types need to calm skin reactivity, you need products and ingredients that turn up the juice. While in their respective chapters, I warn sensitive types *away* from products that are too intense for them, in this chapter, I'll point ORPWs *toward* powerhouse concentrations of active ingredients that your hardy skin calls for.

## A CLOSE-UP LOOK AT YOUR SKIN

If you have ORPW skin, you may experience any of the following:

- Large pores
- Shiny, oily skin
- Trouble finding sunscreen that doesn't make your skin oilier
- Dark spots in sun-exposed areas
- Wrinkles
- Occasional acne breakouts
- Easy use of most skin care and cosmetic products
- Increased risk of skin cancer if you have light skin

I recommend sunscreen for all types, but since you are prone to oiliness, it's essential to find a product that does not increase it. Later in this chapter, I'll offer daily skin care regimens using nonprescription products. Please keep in mind that prescription medications are always more active and therefore most effective. They are particularly important for your skin type.

## HOW YOUR SKIN AGES

ORPW skin changes over time. Younger ORPWs have problems with oil, while older ORPWs lose their oiliness and develop wrinkles. In your fifties your skin may even change to a DRPW Skin Type. That's why using prescription retinoids in your younger years is paramount. These products possess a dual action ideal for you: They help decrease oil secretion *and* prevent wrinkles.

Aging improves oiliness while reducing new dark spots. As your hormone levels drop, so does your production of pigment, causing melasma and dark spots to lessen. However, taking hormone replacement reverses that effect. This is a double bind for ORPWs, since hormone replacement, while worsening pigmentation, helps prevent further wrinkling. I recommend that you consult your gynecologist to make your decision, taking into account both personal and family history.

To prevent and treat both wrinkles and dark spots, I recommend sun avoidance, daily skin care, retinoid use, and other suggestions offered in the procedures section of this chapter. If desired, use self-tanners, which do not worsen dark spots, as some pigmented types fear. Tanners temporarily dye the surface layer of dead skin cells, but don't activate the skin pigments that cause dark spots. To learn more about their use, please see Chapter Ten, "Self-Tanners."

## AN UNDERSERVED SKIN TYPE

For the most part, product researchers and developers fail to formulate products for your special needs. Cosmetic shelves overflow with products for sensitive skin, but none for resistant skin. It's perceived by the industry to be "easy," but with multiple skin problems, yours is not the easiest Resistant Skin Type. Both resistant and oily, your skin's strong barrier keeps out irritating ingredients. The downside is it keeps out *all* ingredients, even beneficial ones your skin needs. That's why it's tough to find nonprescription-strength products that work. Have you ever seen skin care products designed for "tough skin"?

Companies can't regulate who purchases their over-the-counter products. They therefore produce products of lower strength that a sensitive type can safely use because they want to avoid the negative publicity that could result from consumers reacting adversely to their products.

A prescription retinoid is most valuable for ORPW skin because it may decrease oil production and prevent, or even help to eliminate, dark spots and wrinkles. Buy the cheapest cleansers and sunscreens because your resistant skin does not require babying.

For ORPWs, it's definitely worth the expense of an office visit to a dermatologist, who can recommend the powerful prescription medications and medical procedures that will really make a difference. In most cases, insurance will cover your first appointment, and it may very well save you hundreds of dollars that you might have spent on useless skin care products, facials, facial exercising machines, and other minimally effective treatments.

The recommendations I'll offer you will definitely help, but there is no quick fix. Over a lifetime, to help your skin look its best will require dedication, along with the use of retinoids, sunscreen, antioxidants, and the right diet. Your skin's future is up to you.

**Dr. Baumann's Bottom Line:** Go for it! You can use the strongest products. And don't forget to prevent wrinkles by smoking cessation, sun avoidance, and a healthy diet with ample fruits and vegetables.

## EVERYDAY CARE FOR YOUR SKIN TYPE

The goal of your skin care routine is to address dark spots with products that deliver depigmenting ingredients such as kojic acid, arbutin, and hydroquinone and to address wrinkles with products containing retinols and antioxidants. In addition, your daily regimen will help treat oiliness and address blackheads and enlarged pores.

ORPWs who are under thirty will have more problems with oily skin; for those who are older, oil production will have leveled off, but you'll be seeing increased wrinkles. For younger ORPWs, therefore, your goal is to address oiliness and to prevent wrinkles with appropriate skin care. For older ORPWs, wrinkle prevention and treatment is paramount.

In my opinion, no amount of OTC skin care will get rid of wrinkles—you need retinoids or a procedure such as Botox or Juvéderm injections.

If you choose to forgo the prescription route, you can follow the nonprescription regimen indefinitely. In that case, look for toners, sunscreens, facial foundations, and evening treatment lotions or gels that contain retinol, a related but less powerful ingredient. Most retinol products only contain a low amount, so you can safely use several different kinds of skin care products with retinol to increase the results.

## DAILY SKIN CARE

### REGIMEN

#### AM

Step 1: Wash with oil-control cleanser

Step 2: Use toner (optional)

Step 3: Apply skin lightener to spots

Step 4: Apply an oil-control product (optional)

Step 5: Apply moisturizer (optional)

Step 6: Apply sunscreen

Step 7: Apply powder with SPF or oil-absorption qualities

#### PM

Step 1: Wash with glycolic acid or salicylic cleanser

Step 2: Apply skin lightening serum to entire face

Step 3: Apply retinol or antioxidant skin serum

Step 4: Apply moisturizer (optional)

In the morning, wash your face with an oil-control cleanser, then use a toner if you choose. Then apply a skin lightener to dark spots that you wish to treat. Next, you may choose to apply an oil-control product if you have an O/D score over 33. Or if instead you have combination skin (O/D score of 27–33), you can choose to apply a moisturizer in the dry areas (avoid the T-zone). Also, for combination skin, if your face feels slightly dry overall, you can apply moisturizer to your entire face. Then apply a sunscreen. Finally, apply either a powder with SPF or an oil-absorbing powder.

In the evening, wash with a cleanser containing glycolic or salicylic acid. Apply a skin lightening serum to your entire face to help prevent dark spots, then your choice of retinol product or antioxidant serum to help prevent wrinkles. Finally, apply moisturizer if you are using one.

You can also increase exfoliation by using facial scrubs directly after cleansing at night. See the products I recommend later in this section.

# Cleansers

To control oil and prevent enlarged pores, keep your skin clean by using cleansers both morning and evening. ORPWs should stay away from cream cleansers or cold creams. Choose a gel cleanser or a foaming cleanser. Oil-control cleansers and those with glycolic acid and salicylic acid are also good for you.

## RECOMMENDED CLEANSERS

- $   Alpha Hydrox Foaming Face Wash
- $   Neutrogena Oil-Free Acne Wash
- $   Boots Botanics Skin Brightening Deep Clean Gel
- $$   100% Pure Lavender Seafoam Facial Cleanser
- $$   Exuviance Purifying Cleansing Gel
- $$   Joey New York Pure Pores Cleansing Gel w/ Vitamin C
- $$   Lancôme Clarifiance Oil-Free Gel Cleanser
- $$   PCA Skin pHaze 13 Pigment Bar
- $$   Philosophy On a Clear Day Super Wash for Oily Skin
- $$   La Roche-Posay Effaclar Deep Cleansing Foaming Cream
- $$$   N.V. Perricone M.D. Skin Clear Cleanser

**Baumann's Choice:** PCA Skin pHaze 13 Pigment Bar contains lighteners like kojic acid and niacinamide.

# Toner Use

Look for toners with oil-control, depigmenting, and antioxidant ingredients. If using a prescription retinoid, use a toner with alpha hydroxy or beta hydroxy acids. Otherwise, look for a toner with retinol. Those with O/D scores above 33 will probably want to use only a toner and skip the moisturizing step altogether.

## RECOMMENDED TONERS

- $   Boots Botanics Skin Brightening Toner
- $$   La Roche-Posay Effaclar Astringent Lotion
- $$   Rodan & Fields Reverse Prepare Skin Lightening Toner
- $$   SkinCeuticals Equalizing Toner
- $$   YonKa Lotion PNG for Normal to Oily Skin

**Baumann's Choice:** Rodan & Fields Reverse Prepare Skin Lightening Toner if you have dark patches, because it contains hydroquinone and salicylic acid

## Oil-Control Products

You can use an oil-control product in addition to or instead of toners if you have an O/D score of 33 or more. You can also choose oil-control foundations and powders. Blotting tissues are helpful in absorbing oil throughout the day. Many oily types like to keep them handy.

### RECOMMENDED OIL-CONTROL PRODUCTS

$   Seban pads
$$  DDF Glycolic Oil Control Gel
$$  Jack Black Oil Control Lotion
$$  Mary Kay Beauty Blotters Oil-AbsorbingTissues
$$$ Dr. Brandt Pores No More Pore Refiner

**Baumann's Choice:** DDF Glycolic Oil Control Gel because it has glycolic acid

## Treating Dark Spots

For dark spots, use skin lightening products after cleansing and toning, but before other products. Apply at the first sign of a dark spot, and continue until the spot has disappeared completely. To both treat and prevent dark spots, use products containing retinol and other ingredients that increase cell turnover, such as alpha hydroxy and beta hydroxy acids. Niacinamide and soy help prevent the formation of brown spots. Look for soy products that have had the estrogenic components removed (like those from RoC, Neutrogena, and Aveeno). If you find that these nonprescription skin lighteners do not produce results in eight weeks, a dermatologist can prescribe a prescription lightener.

## RECOMMENDED PRODUCTS FOR
## TREATING DARK SPOTS

$   Skineffects by Dr. Jeffrey Dover Advanced Brightening Complex
$$  La Roche-Posay Active C Light
$$  Murad Age Spot & Pigment Lightening Gel
$$  SkinCeuticals Phyto Corrective Gel
$$  Clinique Even Better Clinical Dark Spot Corrector
$$$  Estée Lauder Re-Nutriv Intensive Lifting Serum
$$$  Rodan & Fields Reverse Treatment

**Baumann's Choice:** Rodan & Fields Reverse Treatment because it has hydroquinone and antioxidants

## RECOMMENDED SERUMS TO
## LIGHTEN DARK SPOTS

$   Specific Beauty Skin Brightening Serum
$   Olay Regenerist Daily Regenerating Serum
$$  Murad Age Spot & Pigment Lightening Gel
$$  PCA Skin pHaze 23 A&C Synergy Serum
$$  Philosophy Pigment of Your Imagination Topical Skin Lightener
$$  SkinCeuticals Phyto Corrective Gel
$$$  Rodan & Fields Reverse Treatment

**Baumann's Choice:** PCA Skin pHaze 23 A&C Synergy Serum

## Wrinkle Prevention

Although retinoids are the only effective products for treating wrinkles that have already developed, many OTC products can help *prevent* wrinkles.

## RECOMMENDED ANTIOXIDANT SERUMS
## TO PREVENT WRINKLES

$   Neutrogena Healthy Skin Anti-Wrinkle Lotion
$   Burt's Bees Repair Serum with Attar of Rose
$$  Dr. Andrew Weil for Origins Plantidote Mega-Mushroom Face Serum
$$  La Roche-Posay Active C Light
$$  Laura Mercier Multi Vitamin Serum

$$ SkinCeuticals C E Ferulic
$$$ Alaur Skin Solutions Clock-Stopping C with antioxidants
$$$ Elizabeth Arden Prevage Anti-Aging Treatment
$$$ Combray by Solenne

**Baumann's Choice:** SkinCeuticals C E Ferulic

## Moisturizers

If your O/D score is high (above 35), you probably won't need a moisturizer. With scores of 34 through 44, you may opt to use moisturizer on the dry areas only. If so, look for products formulated for oily skin with oil-control ingredients.

For daytime use, pick a moisturizer with sunscreen. In night creams, search out products with retinol. If you choose to use a moisturizer all over your face—something I recommend only for those with scores between 27 and 33—look for products with lightening ingredients or antioxidants.

### RECOMMENDED MOISTURIZERS

$ Eucerin Q10 Anti-Wrinkle Sensitive Skin Creme
$ Neutrogena Ageless Intensives Deep Wrinkle Anti-Wrinkle Serum
$ RoC Retinol Correxion Deep Wrinkle Night Cream
$ Skineffects by Dr. Jeffrey Dover Daily Anti-Aging Cream with SPF 15
$$ Paula's Choice Skin Balancing Moisture Gel
$$ SkinCeuticals Renew Overnight Oily
$$ Patricia Wexler M.D. Dermatology Skin Brightening Daily Moisturizer SPF 30
$$ YonKa Creme PG
$$$ Murad Energizing Pomegranate Moisturizer SPF 15

**Baumann's Choice:** For AM, Combray is wonderful but it will feel too heavy if you have very oily skin. It is better for slightly oily or combination skin. For very oily skin, I like Patricia Wexler M.D. Dermatology Skin Brightening Daily Moisturizer SPF 30.

For PM, Neutrogena Ageless Intensives Deep Wrinkle Anti-Wrinkle Serum (with retinol, AHAs, and antioxidants)

# Masks

Masks, used once or twice a week, are another good way to give your skin the strong ingredients it needs. I personally think you'd do better going to a spa, salon, or a dermatologist for a chemical peel or microdermabrasion, which can help improve fine lines and dark spots, but if you don't have the time or the money, try a mask. They improve skin oiliness only temporarily, but that can be useful before special occasions, when you want to look your best.

### RECOMMENDED MASKS

- $   Lumene Arctic Touch Deep Cleansing Peat Mask
- $$  Ahava Advanced Mud Masque for Oily Skin
- $$  DDF Clay Mint Mask
- $$  Decleor Aroma Cleanse Clay and Herbal Cleansing Mask
- $$  Elizabeth Arden Deep Cleansing Mask
- $$  Murad Clarifying Mask for Problem Skin
- $$  REN Multi-Mineral Detoxifying Facial Mask
- $$$  Jack Black Deep Detox Clay Mask & Spot Treatment
- $$$  Eminence Lime Stimulating Masque

**Baumann's Choice:** REN Multi-Mineral Detoxifying Facial Mask

# Exfoliation

Cleopatra, famous for her gorgeous skin, was very likely this type. She was known to use sour milk on her face. Without knowing it, she was giving herself a lactic acid–alpha hydroxy acid peel, which speeds the removal of dark spots.

Scrubs and microdermabrasion kits can remove the top, dead layer of the skin to allow better penetration of the active ingredients in toners and moisturizers. If your daily routine includes a prescription retinoid, retinol, alpha hydroxy acid, or beta hydroxy acid product, any form of scrub or exfoliation should be done only twice a week. If you are not using any of these products, you can use your choice of exfoliation product every other day, so long as you don't experience redness or soreness.

Do not use both scrubs and peels; pick one or the other. Too much exfoliation can cause redness and skin sensitivity, making you feel like an OSPW. You can also exfoliate with the Clarisonic MD Skin Care Brush, which has become very popular and is in several colors, including pink.

## RECOMMENDED SCRUBS

$   Bioré Pore Unclogging Scrub

$   Olay Regenerist Detoxifying Pore Scrub

$   Neutrogena Wave Sonic Spinning Power-Cleanser

$$   Vivite Exfoliating Facial Cleanser

$$   Dr. Brandt Microdermabrasion in a Jar

$$   Nia 24 Physical Cleansing Scrub

$$   Philosophy The Microdelivery Peel

$$$   La Prairie Cellular Microdermabrasion Cream

$$$   Clarisonic Skincare Brush

**Baumann's Choice:** Nia 24 Physical Cleansing Scrub because it contains a form of niacinamide

## RECOMMENDED AT-HOME PEEL PRODUCTS

$   Neutrogena Advanced Solutions Facial Peel

$   Olay Regenerist Microdermabrasion & Peel System

$$   Elizabeth Arden Peel & Reveal Revitalizing Treatment

$$   MD Skincare Alpha Beta Daily Face Peel

$$$   AmorePacific Treatment Enzyme Peel

$$$   Natura Bisse Glyco Peeling 50% Pump

**Baumann's Choice:** Alpha Beta Daily Face Peel by MD Skincare, which combines AHA and BHA

## RECOMMENDED KITS

$$   Murad Sun Undone Radiant Skin Renewal Kit

$$   Philosophy Microdelivery Peel

$$$   Obagi System (needs a Retin A prescription to use)

$$$   Rodan & Fields Reverse Regimen

**Baumann's Choice:** Rodan & Fields Reverse Regimen is expensive, but I like the ingredients and it's perfect for your type. If you want to, this is a recommended way to splurge.

## SHOPPING FOR PRODUCTS

To widen your choice of products, read product labels and choose those that contain beneficial ingredients for the particular problem you want to address, as listed below.

There are also ingredients you need to avoid. Some products contain ingredients that can increase oiliness. Others may make your skin more sensitive to sunlight, causing more tanning and dark spots in localized areas. For example, perfumes containing oil of bergamot (also found in Earl Grey tea) can create darkening on the neck. Also, if you drink margaritas while out in the sun, you may notice increased tanning around your mouth or in other areas that come into contact with lime juice.

### RECOMMENDED INGREDIENTS

#### For wrinkle prevention:

- ALA
- Caffeine
- Coenzyme $Q_{10}$ (Ubiquinone)
- Copper peptide
- Ginseng
- Grape seed extract
- Green tea
- Idebenone
- Lutein
- Lycopene
- Moringa
- *Pinus pinaster* (pine bark)
- Pomegranate
- Resveratrol
- Rosemary
- Vitamin C
- Vitamin E

#### For wrinkle treatment:

- Alpha lipoic acid
- Copper peptide
- DMAE
- Glycolic acid (alpha hydroxy acid or AHA)
- Lactic acid
- Phytic acid
- Retinol
- Salicylic acid (beta hydroxy acid, or BHA)
- TGF-Beta

#### To prevent dark spots:

- *Cocos nucifera* (coconut fruit juice)
- Niacinamide

## To hasten removal of dark spots:

- Arbutin
- Bearberry
- Cucumber extract
- *Epilobium angustifolium* (willow herb)
- Gallic acid
- *Glycyrrhiza glabra* (licorice extract)
- Hydroquinone
- Kojic acid
- Mulberry
- Pycnogenol (a pine bark extract)
- Resorcinol
- Retinol
- Salicylic acid (beta hydroxy acid)
- *Saxifraga sarmentosa* extract (strawberry begonia)
- Vitamin C (ascorbic acid)

### SKIN CARE INGREDIENTS TO AVOID

## Due to excess oiliness:

- Mineral oil
- Other oils such as coconut oil
- Petrolatum

## Due to hormonal activity that increases pigmentation and dark spots:

Topical estrogen and estradiol are estrogens present in hormone replacement treatments and some topical creams; these can increase pigmentation. Phytoestrogens, compounds found in plants, also produce similar effects. These include:

- *Cimicifuga racemosa* (black cohosh)
- *Humulus lupulus* (hops)
- Soy (except in Aveeno and Neutrogena products, where the estrogenic ingredient has been removed)
- *Trifolium pretense* (red clover)
- *Vitex agnus-castus* (chasteberry)
- Wild yams

*Due to skin darkening effects:*

- Extracts of celery, limes, parsley, figs, and carrots
- Oil of bergamot

## Sun Protection for Your Skin

Most sunscreens are formulated in an oil base because their active ingredients are usually oil-soluble. Oily sunscreens can make your skin look shiny, so use gels or sprays. Powders with SPF are another excellent option. One of my favorites is a powder foundation with sunscreen (SPF 15) made by Philosophy that's called The Supernatural. Formulated for oily skin, it comes in two shades to match different skin tones.

Sunscreens have greatly improved in the United States since the FDA approved Helioplex and Mexoryl—two superior UVA protective ingredients. Mexoryl can be found in Vichy and La Roche-Posay products. Helioplex is in Neutrogena products. Aveeno also contains Helioplex, but they call it "active photobarrier complex." Look for sunscreens that contain these ingredients.

### RECOMMENDED SUN PROTECTION PRODUCTS

- $ Aveeno Continuous Sunblock Lotion for the face SPF 30
- $ Neutrogena Ultra Sheer Dry-Touch Sunblock SPF 100+
- $ Eucerin Q10 Anti-Wrinkle Sensitive Skin Lotion SPF 15
- $$ Exuviance Fundamental Multi-Protective Day Fluid SPF 15
- $$ Glycolix Elite Sunscreen SPF 30 by Glycolix Elite
- $$ La Roche-Posay Anthelios 60 Ultra Light Sunscreen Fluid Extreme, SPF 60
- $$ Neostrata Oil-Free Lotion SPF 15
- $$ Olay Age Defying Anti-Wrinkle Daily SPF 15 Lotion
- $$ RevaléSkin CoffeeBerry Day Cream SPF 15

**Baumann's Choice:** La Roche-Posay, Neutrogena, or Aveeno purchased after June 2010

## Your Makeup

ORPWs may have trouble choosing makeup foundations. To cover dark spots, you need a heavier foundation, which may streak. If you're over forty, heavier makeup products can run into wrinkles, making them more noticeable.

If pigment is not a problem, choose a sheerer foundation and cover it with a powder. If pigment is a problem, choose a heavier foundation that hides dark spots and also works well for oily skin, such as Exuviance Cover-Blend Concealing Treatment Makeup SPF 20.

Since you can never get enough sunscreen, use makeup products containing SPF whenever you can. Also listed below are a concealer and lip color that both have sunscreen.

### RECOMMENDED FOUNDATIONS

$  Revlon Colorstay for Combo/Oily Skin Makeup with SoftFlex SPF 6

$$  Bobbi Brown Oil-Free Even Finish Foundation SPF 15

$$  Exuviance CoverBlend Concealing Treatment Makeup SPF 20

$$  Laura Mercier Oil-Free Foundation

$$$  Lancôme Teint Idole Fresh Wear

**Baumann's Choice:** All are good.

### RECOMMENDED POWDERS

$  Neutrogena Healthy Skin Pressed Powder Compact SPF 20

$  Paula's Select Healthy Finish Pressed Powder with SPF 15

$$  Almay TLC Truly Lasting Color Pressed Powder SPF 12

$$  Philosophy The Supernatural Airbrushed Canvas

$$  Physician's Formula Healthy Wear SPF 50 Powder Foundation

$$$  Diorskin Nude Natural Glow Sculpting Powder Makeup SPF 10

**Baumann's Choice:** Visitors to the ORPW forum at www.skintype solutions.com rave about the Physician's Formula Healthy Wear SPF 50 Powder Foundation. My patients love it too!

You can make your makeup needs work for you. Look for a powder compact that can also be a fashion statement. I have dry skin and do not use much facial powder; however, I have a passion for collecting powder compacts. I have vintage ones, gorgeous new ones by Jay Strongwater and look forward every Christmas to the new compacts by Estée Lauder. I have to admit that I'm addicted to shopping for powder compacts on eBay. For those of you with oily skin, carry one of the gorgeous compacts with you and touch up your makeup every few hours or before a photograph to prevent the telltale oily signs.

## PROCEDURES FOR YOUR SKIN TYPE

Procedures like lasers and light treatments can't be used on dark skin. Instead, ORPWs with dark skin tones can use topical products to decrease oiliness and dark spots. Resistant types have an advantage over sensitive types, because you can use stronger ingredients without fear of sensitivity, so you may see results faster. Expect to wait about four to eight weeks to see the dark spots improve. Dark-skinned ORPWs may also benefit from chemical peels containing salicylic acid (BHA) 20 percent or 30 percent or combinations of glycolic acid and other depigmenting ingredients. Prescription retinoids used in your skin care regimen will enhance the penetration of the peel and will help you heal faster afterward by stepping up cell division.

If you have darker skin, choose a dermatologist who is skilled at treating dark-skinned people, because dark spots can worsen if chemical peels are not done correctly. These peels range from $120 to $250 per peel, and a series of five to eight is normal.

### To Reduce Pores

Skin care procedures such as facials and microdermabrasion don't really decrease pore size. However, you can obtain temporary pore reduction by using products containing AHAs, BHA, and vitamin C as recommended in the nonprescription product section.

### To Reduce Oiliness

For those with light skin, light procedures, such as IPL procedures with Levulan, may decrease oil secretion by shrinking the oil-producing glands.

## Procedures to Treat Wrinkles

A number of procedures are available to treat wrinkles. They include injections of botulinum toxin (Botox or Reloxin) and dermal fillers. Lasers and other forms of light treatment for wrinkles show promise for the future, but they are not yet indisputedly effective. In addition, there is a new technique called Titan. ORPWs are ideal candidates for it.

## ONGOING CARE FOR YOUR SKIN

Avoid the sun and stop smoking to preserve your skin. Plus, use retinols and retinoids to reverse sun damage and the signs of aging. Eat an antioxidant-rich diet. If your pocketbook will permit, go for procedures that will bring real results. Your resistant, pigmented skin will help protect you from the side effects that other types develop after these procedures. The latest technology is there for you!

# CHAPTER NINE

# Oily, Resistant, Pigmented, and Tight: ORPT

## BAUMANN SKIN TYPE NUMBER 9

■

*"I want to brighten and even my complexion. I have few or no wrinkles, but I am confused about what moisturizers and sunscreens are best for my skin. Do I need a toner? Many creams feel too heavy. I need a regimen that works for my skin type."*

### ABOUT YOUR SKIN

Yours is definitely one of the easier Skin Types, since your type's strengths far outweigh its deficits. Oily, resistant, and tight skin looks great and ages well. Yes, you may get acne (especially in youth) and some dark spots, but your easy care skin has a vibrancy and glow that many ORPTs take for granted.

Luckily, you rarely develop the stinging, redness, or product allergies often experienced by more sensitive types. Oily skin is troublesome in youth but, for women, will often improve with menopause. The dark spots, which are your nemesis, do have an upside: The pigmentation that causes them also protects you from skin cancer. Finally, tight skin helps you retain your youthful appearance when other types are hunting down antiaging remedies. Your skin is to be coveted and also protected with regular sunscreen use (even if you have dark-toned skin) as well as a diet high in antioxidant-rich fruits and vegetables.

ORPT skin is quite common among people with a darker skin color like the many Caribbean Americans I see in my Florida practice. Lighter-skin-toned people from other ethnic backgrounds, like the Irish, English, and others, can also be ORPTs. So can a redhead with freckles, which are a form of pigmentation. That's why if the questionnaire revealed that you're an ORPT, but you don't experience all the symptoms I'll cover, you shouldn't worry that your result is wrong. All ORPTs share a number of common problems, but there are some significant differences, so throughout this chapter, I'll discuss the range of symptoms and tendencies, as well as the various treatment options, available to dark-, medium-, and light-toned ORPTs.

## SKIN COLOR AND THE ORPT

The recommendations in this chapter will help your skin glow more vibrantly, whether you are a dark-skinned ORPT or a light-skinned one. While anyone can have this Skin Type, a high proportion of ORPTs are African Americans, Latin Americans, Mediterraneans, and Asians. By the way, even though Asian skin may look light, it often reacts similarly to darker skin. If you have Asian ancestry, consider yourself in the dark-skinned ORPT group, which will affect the skin recommendations you follow later in this chapter.

I've found that light-toned ORPTs generally have both good genes and healthy skin habits that protect them from the ravages of aging. They often eat lots of fruits and vegetables, do not smoke, and do not intentionally seek sun exposure. I say: Good for you, as this combination helps to prevent wrinkles. For others reading this chapter, if you'd like to prevent wrinkles too, remember, genes tell only part of the story, and lifestyle factors can make a big difference!

## YOUR SKIN ISSUES

All dark-skinned ORPTs readily develop dark spots, triggered by any form of skin injury or inflammation, including cuts, burns, bruises, and scrapes. Allergic reactions are less common for you than for sensitive types. In most cases, stronger topical products can easily prevent or lighten them, so thank your resistant skin that you can use them while sensitive types cannot. Ingrown hairs can cause dark spots, and dark-skinned male ORPTs experience this in the beard area, especially if they shave.

Women may have excessive facial hair above the lip, on the cheeks, or elsewhere. Darker-skin-toned ORPTs have darker-colored hair, making unwanted hair growth more noticeable. However, hair removal can create further problems: Waxing and chemical depilatories can irritate your skin and leave dark spots in their wake. Plucking hairs can lead to tweezer injury, subsequently leaving dark spots.

Your second major issue is acne and facial shine. You may battle with oily skin, struggle with troublesome breakouts, despair that your face always looks shiny in photos, and avoid wearing necessary sun protection because you can't stand its greasy feel. The trick is to find a sunscreen and other products that don't add to your skin's innate oiliness.

In order to smooth and soften, products like hair conditioners often include ingredients that remain after washing. They're good for your hair, but a big problem for your skin. Always wash your face after washing and conditioning your hair to remove all product residue. You should also be cautious with bug sprays, sunscreens, hair gels, leave-in conditioners, hand lotions, and other products that may come into contact with your face, as they can contribute to greasiness.

Finding products that fight oil and inflammation without adding oil, or triggering brown spots, is essential. Certain ingredients widely included in skin care stimulate hormones like estrogen that activate pigmentation, thereby contributing to the formation of brown spots. That's where my ingredient lists will help. I'll offer you my recommendations for a daily routine with a selection of products most effective for ORPT skin. If you're inclined to shop and experiment, check ingredients, and make sure to avoid those that are "estrogenic," like the ones I detail in the "Shopping for Products" section of this chapter.

In the past, some products may have backfired because of the combination of issues you must address. Others may not have been effective enough to help your sturdy and resistant skin. It's a matter of finding the right balance.

## A CLOSE-UP LOOK AT YOUR SKIN

ORPTs typically have minimal skin problems; if they use poor products or, worse, think their skin can take care of itself in all situations, they may experience oiliness or acne.

With either dark, medium, or light ORPT skin, you may experience any of the following:

- Face looks shiny, especially in photographs
- Facial foundation streaks
- Sunscreens feel oily
- Dark spots develop on face

- Skin tans easily
- Minimal facial wrinkles
- Occasional acne breakouts

Whatever your skin color, I don't recommend tanning or excess sun exposure and I do recommend regular sunscreen use for all ORPTs. Even though you probably look gorgeous tanned, resist the urge, and use self-tanners. You'll thank me later! (For instructions on their use, please refer to "Self-Tanners" in Chapter Ten.)

## DARK-SKINNED ORPTs

When I surveyed my black patients, I found that few wore sunscreen, assuming that they did not need it. People with darker skin tones do have some built-in protection from the sun, but dark pigmentation alone won't prevent dark spots. I see proof of that every day, as many of my patients are people of color, and the most common reason they come to see me is for help in treating their dark spots.

Beyond its role in activating the pigment production that triggers dark spots, excess sun exposure can also have other harmful effects. When you get too much sun, your body temporarily suppresses your immune system's response mechanisms for anywhere from a day to three days. As a result, for a few days following sun exposure, you may be more vulnerable to colds and flu, which is why some people get summer colds. (Obviously, winter colds in colder climes are due to other factors.) Viral infections, like herpes, may also occur more easily due to this temporary immunosuppression.

The bottom line is that sun protection should be a priority for everyone, regardless of skin color or tone. And sunscreen should be used on a daily—not a sporadic—basis.

Finding the right color of sunscreen, facial powder, and foundation can be a problem for darker-skin-toned people. For example, there are over two hundred different shades of Asian skin, but as far as I know, no company offers two hundred shades of makeup foundation! While often oily types dislike the greasy feel of sun products, many dark-skinned people find that creamy white products turn their skin a violet or whitish color. Finding the right moisturizer is also key. Luckily, several tinted moisturizers are now available as companies recognize the need to develop skin care products geared to dark-skinned people.

With dark ORPT skin, you may experience any of the following:

- Dark spots in areas of previous irritation
- Shiny face, especially with sunscreen use
- White or purple skin hues when using sunscreens
- Difficulty finding the right color of facial foundation
- Streaking of facial foundations
- Ingrown hairs with resulting dark spots
- Dark circles under the eyes

## LIGHT-SKINNED ORPTs

Like dark-skinned ORPTs, light-skinned ORPTs will tend to develop dark spots. But in your case, they will most likely be freckles. As a consequence, you may have learned to avoid the sun. Remember in *Gone with the Wind* when Scarlett O'Hara was applying buttermilk to her shoulders to get rid of freckles from the sun? She was probably a light-skinned ORPT! (Do you think the real-life Southern belles knew that buttermilk contains lactic acid, an alpha hydroxy acid that helps remove dark spots by increasing exfoliation?)

ORPTs with light skin have it easier than those with dark skin for several reasons. Your freckles and sun spots can be greatly improved by laser and light treatments. Dark-skinned people's higher levels of melanin absorb too much of the laser or light energy, which damages the normal skin in the area.

If you have light ORPT skin, you may experience:

- Shiny face, especially with sunscreen use
- Freckling on face and body
- Sun spots on hands, arms, and legs
- Increased risk for melanoma skin cancer, especially if you have red hair

## THE DOWNSIDE OF TIGHT SKIN

Those of you with the ORPT Type may have genes on your side, but that doesn't make you immune to bad skin care habits. For example, let's take two people with similar but slightly different types, such as an ORPT (like you) and an ORPW. While excess sun and smoking will not cause wrinkles as much for your T skin, they will increase the likelihood of skin cancer, especially in light-skinned ORPTs, who are already at risk. Also, bad skin habits can cause you to revert to a W type. This is one skin factor that you can significantly control, so good habits are important. (See Chapter Two for more on tightness vs. wrinkling.)

Since light-skinned ORPTs are at higher risk of melanoma skin cancer, it's essential to wear sunscreen consistently, especially when out in the sun. This type of skin cancer is the most deadly kind, and that's why I urge all Pigmented, Tight Skin Types to make certain to check on anything suspicious. If you have fair skin, red hair, and freckles, please get annual skin exams to search for melanoma, which is completely curable when caught early.

## The A, B, C, and D of Melanoma

Four things to look out for include:

1. Asymmetry: One side of the mole is not a mirror image of the other side.
2. Borders: The borders are not distinct. It is hard to tell where the mole starts and stops.
3. Color: The presence of more than one color, or black, white, red, and yellow hues
4. Diameter: Greater than or equal to the size of a pencil eraser

If you have moles with any of these characteristics, see a dermatologist immediately. If you or your family have a history of melanoma, make an appointment for a routine skin exam every six months. Insurance should cover these visits. If you are redheaded, Australian, or have a history of many sunburns, you are also at an increased risk of developing melanoma.

## AGING AND THE ORPT

As you get older, your skin problems will likely decrease. The exception is that you may develop more sun spots if you have light skin and are prone to them. Most ORPTs enjoy their skin during their fifties and sixties, the decades of life when other types are reaching for wrinkle creams or are running for plastic surgery.

You're lucky for several reasons. First, as you go through menopause, oil secretion tends to decrease. Second, estrogen levels (contributing to dark spots and melasma) will decline with age, causing those problems to improve. Hormonal fluctuations caused by pregnancy, birth control pill use, and perimenopause stabilize. Of course, if you opt to take hormone replacement therapy, you may continue to suffer from dark spots. People with dry, wrinkled skin may experience some improvement on hormone replacement therapy (HRT), but neither of these is a problem for you. Deciding for or against HRT is a decision to be made in consultation with your gynecologist, along with an assessment of family history and other risk factors. But overall, ORPT skin has no compelling need for it.

**Dr. Baumann's Bottom Line:** Enjoy your glowing skin, but don't take it for granted! Following my Daily Skin Care Regimen and other recommendations will help assure that your ORPT skin remains low maintenance and problem free. The right habits, like sunscreen use, smoking cessation, and getting plenty of antioxidants, will assure you youthful skin for a lifetime. Protect your skin and it will protect you.

## EVERYDAY CARE FOR YOUR SKIN TYPE

The goal of your skin care routine is to address oiliness and brown spots, with oil-control products, bleaching ingredients, and ingredients that help prevent dark spots.

Your skin can handle strong bleaching agents. I'll be recommending products that are strong enough to be effective yet are not heavy or greasy, so they don't make your skin look oilier.

Dark spots are your number-one skin problem. Although some ORPTs are not bothered by oily skin, others are. I'll provide a two-part regimen: one part to get rid of the dark spots, and one for maintenance, to prevent them from coming back. Try the two-part over-the-counter protocol first for eight weeks, and then, if it does not work, see your dermatologist. While nonprescription products are not quite as strong as prescription ones, they can sometimes be effective in lightening dark spots, and they often contain additional ingredients that help improve acne. However, since your resistant skin can handle the high percentages of active ingredients in the prescription medications, I suggest you go for it—use the prescription meds. Unfortunately, most of these medications will not be covered by insurance. But the chances are that your insurance will at least cover your office visit to get the prescriptions.

## DAILY SKIN CARE

---

### REGIMEN FOR GETTING RID OF DARK SPOTS:

| AM | PM |
|---|---|
| Step 1: Wash with cleanser | Step 1: Wash with same cleanser as in AM |
| Step 2: Apply a glycolic acid product, such as toner or at-home peel | Step 2: Apply a skin lightener to spots |
| Step 3: Apply sunscreen | Step 3: Apply retinol-containing product |
| Step 4: Apply oil-absorbing powder or powder with SPF | |

---

In the morning, use a cleanser to clean your face, then apply a glycolic acid face toner or peel. Next, apply sunscreen. Last, apply a powder, if desired. Many companies are now launching cosmetics with a range of colors suited to both light- and dark-skinned ORPTs.

In the evening, wash with the same cleanser that you used in the morning, then apply a skin lightener to dark spots. Last, apply a moisturizer containing retinol. This will help to control oil and prevent future brown spots, while also providing basic wrinkle prevention. Eye creams and serums, which are optional for your type, can be applied prior to sunscreen application in your morning protocol, and prior to moisturizer application in your evening protocol.

If you choose to try this regimen, continue it for eight weeks. If you find that it successfully eliminates the dark spots on your skin, move to the nonprescription maintenance regimen on the following page to prevent new dark spots from occurring.

If this regimen does not successfully get rid of your dark spots after eight weeks, it's time to see your dermatologist.

## REGIMEN FOR PREVENTING DARK SPOTS:

| AM | PM |
|---|---|
| Step 1: Wash with cleanser | Step 1: Wash with same cleanser as in AM |
| Step 2: Apply glycolic acid toner or peel product | Step 2: Apply a retinol-containing product |
| Step 3: Apply sunscreen | |

In the morning, wash your face with a cleanser, then use a facial peel, or toner if preferred. Next, apply sunscreen. If skin feels oily, you can also opt to use a facial powder that contains SPF.

In the evening, clean your face with the same cleanser that you used in the morning, then apply a retinol product for ongoing oil control, wrinkle, and dark-spot prevention.

Eye creams and serums, which are optional for your type, can be applied prior to sunscreen application in your morning protocol, and prior to moisturizer application in your evening protocol.

## RECOMMENDED CLEANSING PRODUCTS

$ Aveeno Positively Radiant Cleansing Pads
$ Alpha Hydrox Foaming Face Wash Clarifying Cleanser
$$ La Roche-Posay Effaclar Foaming Purifying Gel
$$ M.D. Forté Facial Cleanser II
$$ MD Formulations Facial Cleanser
$$ Peter Thomas Roth Glycolic Acid 3% Facial Wash
$$ Philosophy Purity Made Simple Facial Cleanser
$$ Vivite Exfoliating Cleanser
$$ SkinCeuticals Simply Clean Pore-Refining Cleanser
$$$ Boscia Purifying Cleansing Gel
$$$ Dr. Brandt Pores No More Cleanser
$$$ Estée Lauder Sparkling Clean Purifying Mud Foam Cleanser

**Baumann's Choice:** Aveeno Positively Radiant Cleansing Pads with soy to help prevent dark spots. The estrogenic components of the soy have been taken out.

## Toner Use

You can use toners that contain ingredients that control oil production, absorb oil, exfoliate, or lighten dark spots.

### RECOMMENDED TONER PRODUCTS

- $    Burt's Bees Garden Tomato Toner for Oily and Troubled Skin
- $$    Gly Derm Solution 5% (contains glycolic acid)
- $$    La Roche-Posay Effaclar Astringent Lotion
- $$    L'Occitane Brightening Water
- $$$    Lancôme Tonique Radiance Clarifying Exfoliating Toner

**Baumann's Choice:** Gly Derm Solution 5% because it contains glycolic acid, which will help exfoliate

## Oil-Control Products

These products offer options for on-the-spot oil control that you can use on an as-needed basis at any time.

### RECOMMENDED OIL-CONTROL PRODUCTS

- $    The Body Shop Tea Tree Oil Facial Blotting Tissues
- $    Mary Kay Beauty Blotters Oil-Absorbing Tissues
- $$    DDF Glycolic Oil Control Gel
- $$$    Origins Zero Oil

**Baumann's Choice:** DDF Glycolic Oil Control Gel because it has glycolic acid

## Treating Dark Spots

If you have dark spots, you can use skin lightening products on them, making sure to use them after cleansing and toning but before other recommended products. Start using the products at the first sign of a dark spot, and continue them until it has completely disappeared. If these nonprescription skin lighteners are not effective enough, consult a dermatologist, who can prescribe a prescription lightener.

In addition, you can use products containing retinol that increase the rate of cell turnover to prevent brown spots from occurring. Use these nonprescription retinol-containing gels and moisturizers alone when no brown spots are present and with a spot-removing toner or gel containing ingredients that decrease brown spots when spots are present.

### RECOMMENDED RETINOL-CONTAINING PRODUCTS

*To treat and prevent brown spots:*

- $ Black Opal Essential Fade Complex
- $ RoC Retinol Correxion Deep Wrinkle Daily Moisturizer SPF 30
- $$ Afirm 3x
- $$ La Roche-Posay Biomedic Retinol Cream 60
- $$ PCA Skin pHaze 23 A&C Synergy Serum
- $$ Philosophy Help Me (with retinol)
- $$ Replenix Retinol Smoothing Serum 5x by Topix
- $$$ SkinCeuticals Retinol 1.0

**Baumann's Choice:** All are good.

## Skin Lightening Kits

You're lucky because there are a number of product lines developed especially for you, and some of these prepackaged kits are a good choice.

### RECOMMENDED SKIN CARE KITS FOR DARK SPOTS

- $$$ Regenerist Microdermabrasion & Peel System
- $$$ Obagi NuDerm (This six-step program takes longer to apply than the others, but the time spent may be worthwhile for resistant types. A prescription retinoid is required for the fifth step.)
- $$$ Rodan & Fields Reverse Regimen (This four-step kit from the makers of Proactiv contains cleanser, toner, bleaching gel, and sunscreen. Although the sunscreen is white, it absorbs quickly and does not look white or violet on darker skin.)

**Baumann's Choice:** I like them all.

## Moisturizers

Regular moisturizer use is unnecessary and can make the skin appear more oily. However, in a dry, cold, or windy climate, use a moisturizer to protect your skin. If you have dark spots, look for moisturizers that contain soy, niacinamide, mulberry, kojic acid, hydroquinone, or licorice extract. In the morning, apply one with SPF or apply a sunscreen over your moisturizer.

For dark circles under your eyes, use eye creams containing retinol and vitamin K.

### RECOMMENDED MOISTURIZERS

- $ Aveeno Positively Radiant Daily Moisturizer with SPF
- $ Eucerin Everyday Protection Face Lotion SPF 30
- $ Neutrogena Healthy Skin Anti-Wrinkle Cream (original formula)
- $ Olay Total Effects 7x Visible Anti-Aging Vitamin Complex
- $ RoC Retinol Correxion Deep Wrinkle Night Cream
- $ Skin Effects Preventing Effects Lightweight Moisturizing Souffle Spf 30+
- $$ SkinCeuticals Renew Overnight Oily
- $$ Nia 24 Intensive Recovery Complex
- $$ YonKa Creme PG
- $$ Vivite Daily Facial Moisturizer with Sunscreen SPF 30

**Baumann's Choice:** Vivite Daily Facial Moisturizer with Sunscreen SPF 30 because it contains glycolic acid and a sunscreen

### RECOMMENDED EYE CREAMS AND SERUMS

- $ Olay Regenerist Eye Lifting Serum
- $$ Quintessence Clarifying Under-Eye Serum
- $$ Murad Lighten and Brighten Eye Treatment

**Baumann's Choice:** Quintessence Clarifying Under-Eye Serum—combines vitamin K and retinol

# Masks

Masks, used once or twice a week, can give your skin the strong ingredients it needs. You're better off going to a spa, salon, or dermatologist for a chemical peel or microdermabrasion. These treatments help improve fine lines and dark spots. But if you don't have the time or the money, try the products listed below. They improve skin oiliness only temporarily, but are helpful for special occasions.

### RECOMMENDED MASKS

$ Alba Hawaiian Facial Mask, Papaya Enzyme
$$ Zia Natural Skincare Fresh Papaya Enzyme Mask
$$ DDF Sulfur Therapeutic Mask
$$ Gly Derm Gly Masque 3%
$$ Jurlique Moor Purifying Mask
$$ Laura Mercier Deep Cleansing Clay Mask
$$ MD Formulations Vit-A-Plus Clearing Complex Masque
$$ Murad Clarifying Mask for Problem Skin
$$$ Astara Blue Flame Purification Mask
$$$ Jan Marini Factor A Plus Mask

**Baumann's Choice:** Gly Derm Gly Masque 3% with glycolic acid

# Facial Peels

Although these peels are lower in strength than what you can get at a salon or spa, if used on daily basis, they do convey some benefits.

### RECOMMENDED FACIAL PEELS

$ Soap & Glory The Fab Pore Facial Peel
$ 100% Pure Facial Peel, Pineapple Enzyme Facial Peel
$$ Elizabeth Arden Peel & Reveal Revitalizing Treatment
$$ MD Skincare Alpha Beta Daily Face Peel
$$ Vichy Microabrasion Peel
$$ skyn Iceland Nordic Skin Peel with biospheric complex
$$$ Natura Bisse Glyco Peeling 50% Pump

**Baumann's Choice:** Vichy Microabrasion Peel—check www.skintype solutions.com for other favorites

## Exfoliation

You can benefit from gentle exfoliation, but no more than two to three times a week. Overdoing it can cause inflammation and lead to dark spots, especially if you have darker skin. You can also purchase a Clarisonic MD Skin Care system from your dermatologist.

### RECOMMENDED EXFOLIATORS

- $ Buf-Puf
- $ St. Ives Naturally Clear Green Tea Scrub
- $ Specific Beauty Exfoliating Cleansing Cloths
- $ St. Ives Swiss Formula Invigorating Apricot Scrub
- $$ DDF Pumice Acne Scrub
- $$ Dermalogica Skin Prep Scrub
- $$$ Dr. Brandt Microdermabrasion in a Jar

**Baumann's Choice:** Specific Beauty Exfoliating Cleansing Cloths

## SHOPPING FOR PRODUCTS

Widen your choice of products by reading labels to select products with beneficial ingredients and avoid ones that tend to cause pigmentation or oiliness. Certain food extracts such as lemon or lime (and essential oils, like oil of bergamot) may make skin more sensitive to sunlight, resulting in increased tanning and dark spots. People enjoying margaritas while sitting in the sun may notice darkened skin in areas that are splashed by lime juice. Ingredients with "estrogenic effects" may worsen hormone-related dark spots such as melasma. If you find products that you like that are not on the list of recommendations, please go to www.skintypesolutions.com and share them with me.

## SKIN CARE INGREDIENTS TO USE

### For getting rid of dark spots:

- Arbutin
- Bearberry extract
- Cucumber extract
- *Glycyrrhiza glabra* (licorice extract)
- Hydroquinone
- Kojic acid
- Mulberry extract
- Niacinamide
- Retinol
- Salicylic acid (beta hydroxy acid)
- Vitamin C (ascorbic acid)

### To speed up skin renewal:

- Beta hydroxy acid (salicylic acid)
- Retinaldehyde
- Retinol

### Alpha hydroxy acids such as:

- Citric acid
- Glycolic acid
- Lactic acid
- Phytic acid

## SKIN CARE INGREDIENTS TO AVOID

### Due to skin darkening:

- Extracts of celery, lemon, lime, parsley, fig, and carrot
- Oil of bergamot

### Due to estrogenic effects, increasing pigmentation levels:

- Genistein
- Soy, except when found in Aveeno, RoC, and Neutrogena products (in which estrogenic fractions have been removed)
- Topical estrogen (such as estradiol)

## Sun Protection for Your Skin

Make sure to use sunscreen to prevent dark spots. Even if you have very dark skin, it's a must! Cream sunscreens can make your skin appear even oilier and will increase makeup streaking. That's why most ORPTs prefer powders and gels. Powder sunscreens are perfect for your type because they absorb oil but do not rely on them for sun protection. Dark-skinned patients may dislike the whiteness of sunscreens. This will often disappear after a few minutes. If it does not, look for a tinted sunscreen.

### RECOMMENDED SUN PROTECTION PRODUCTS

- $ Aveeno Positively Radiant Daily Moisturizer with SPF
- $ mark Get A Tint Tinted Moisturizer Lotion SPF 15
- $ Specific Beauty Daily Hydrating Lotion SPF 30
- $ Neutrogena Healthy Powder
- $ Skineffects by Dr. Jeffrey Dover Daily Anti-Aging Cream with SPF 15
- $$ La Roche-Posay Anthelios 60 Ultra Light Sunscreen Fluid Extreme, SPF 60
- $$ Mary Kay TimeWise Day Solution with Sunscreen SPF 15
- $$ Philosophy A Pigment of Your Imagination SPF 18 Sunscreen
- $$ SkinCeuticals Daily Sun Defense SPF 20
- $$$ Nia24 Sun Damage Prevention 100% Mineral Sunscreen SPF 30

**Baumann's Choice:** Specific Beauty Daily Hydrating Lotion SPF 30. It was designed by my colleague Dr. Heather Woolery-Lloyd specifically for multi-hued and darker skin tones.

## Your Makeup

Makeup can cover dark spots, but many foundations streak on oily skin. Instead use powders and powder-based foundations. You can also use a foundation and apply a powder on top of it. Look for products that have sunscreen (you can never have too much). Some new facial foundations contain ingredients such as soy that help lighten dark spots.

If oiliness and streaking are your main problems, stay away from liquid foundations; use tinted sunscreens instead and cover them with an oil-control powder. Use these powders dry and apply with a puff to reduce shine.

## RECOMMENDED FOUNDATIONS

$    Iman Second To None Oil-Free Makeup SPF 8 (for darker-
     skinned people)
$    Revlon ColorStay Makeup with SoftFlex SPF 6
$$   Bobbi Brown Oil-Free Even Finish Foundation SPF 15
$$$  Tarte Smooth Operator SPF 20

**Baumann's Choice:** Revlon ColorStay Makeup with SoftFlex SPF 6

## RECOMMENDED FACIAL POWDERS

$    CoverGirl Fresh Complexion Pocket Powder
$    Neutrogena Healthy Skin Pressed Powder Compact SPF 20
$    Maybelline Shine Free Oil-Control Pressed Powder
$$   Bobbi Brown Sheer Finish Loose Powder
$$   Laura Mercier Foundation Powder
$$   Clinique Stay-Matte Sheer Pressed Powder
$$$  Shu Uemura Face Powder Matte

**Baumann's Choice:** CoverGirl Fresh Complexion Pocket Powder

## PROCEDURES FOR YOUR SKIN TYPE

Dark-skinned ORPTs usually find that topical products are effective for
eliminating dark spots, which means you can avoid the more costly, unnecessary, and sometime harmful procedures. But be patient, as topical products will take some time before showing results.

## Light Treatments

For those with light skin, light procedures, such as IPL procedures with
Levulan, may decrease oil secretion by shrinking the oil-producing glands.
If your skin is medium-dark to dark, I advise against light treatments be-
cause they can lead to inflammation and worsen dark spots.

## Chemical Peels

Chemical peels are an option for those with darker skin tones, or for those who want to stay clear of expensive IPLs. Your dermatologist can perform facial peels with AHAs and BHA in strengths higher than you can find in an over-the-counter product or in spas. These peels contain salicylic acid (BHA) 20 percent or 30 percent, or combinations of glycolic acid and other depigmenting ingredients. I strongly recommend asking your dermatologist about the PCA Peel and Jessner's peel, which are perfect for you. However, if you prefer to go to a spa, ask for peels such as glycolic acid or a modified Jessner's peel.

If you have darker skin, make certain that you go to a dermatologist who is skilled at treating people with similar skin—dark spots can worsen if chemical peels are done incorrectly. Peels range from $120 to $250 per peel; a series of five to eight is usually recommended.

## Microdermabrasion

Microdermabrasion may help spots disappear faster as well. Dark-skinned people should be extra cautious about getting treatments from anyone other than a dermatologist. Treatments that are too strong can worsen your spots.

## Reducing Pores

Neither skin care products, facials, microdermabrasion, nor cosmetics can decrease the size of your pores. Any decrease you might observe is caused by ingredients in the products making the skin surrounding the pores swell slightly, so the pores temporarily appear to shrink. Instead, try using products containing AHAs and BHA and vitamin C. These may help reduce pore size, though only temporarily.

## ONGOING CARE FOR YOUR SKIN

By following my oil-decreasing and pigment-prevention regimens, you can get the most out of your easy-care skin. Be thankful you have one of the easier Skin Types, and bask in the glow!

# CHAPTER TEN

# Oily, Resistant, Non-Pigmented, and Wrinkled: ORNW

## BAUMANN SKIN TYPE NUMBER 12

■

*"My skin feels oilier in the summer, especially when it is humid. I rarely get irritated from skin care products, but I also find that few products work well for me all year long. Please help me understand how to adjust my skin care regimen to ensure that I am using all the proper ingredients to prevent skin aging."*

## ABOUT YOUR SKIN

Your skin is so easy, you haven't focused on it. Since the majority of Americans have your Skin Type, most skin care products, like drugstore toners or face soaps, are geared to you, so they seem to work just fine. Unlike sensitive types, your skin can withstand a wide range of chemicals without experiencing irritation or redness. As a result, you can use any skin care item without worry. When others fuss over skin care, you can't imagine why. You take your skin for granted.

Unlike pigmented types, you don't need to contend with dark spots. Unlike dry types, your need to moisturize is minimal, and until you age, greasy creams hold no appeal. Although you experienced some pimples and oiliness during your teen years, this too seemed perfectly normal. You could handle it with a drugstore pimple treatment product, just like everyone else.

Sunscreen? You probably didn't bother with it. Most sunscreens felt greasy, and a little sun is good for acne, you heard somewhere. If you burned occasionally, so what? So did everyone else. The problem with

ORNW skin is that most of your skin problems hit you late in life, and you're not prepared for them. Wrinkles, sags, and other signs of aging seem to appear overnight. You're caught off guard, because you're used to easy skin care. When aging happens to *you,* its effects aren't so pretty. You never thought it could happen, but now when you look in the mirror, you worry—just like everyone else.

## CARING FOR YOUR SKIN

Controlling oiliness is your goal before the age of forty, while addressing wrinkles will be your goal thereafter. ORNWs gravitate to facials to clear the pimples, blackheads, and whiteheads common to oily skin. Although facials are too drying or irritating for many other types, Oily, Resistant Skin Types are free to enjoy them. One tip: look for a facial that uses products rich in antioxidant ingredients, which help prevent wrinkles.

Don't permit your facialist to extract your blackheads or whiteheads, which can lead to scarring. Nor should you squeeze them at home. Always resist the urge. Use a cleanser with salicylic acid or adhesive strips such as Bioré to gently clean the pores instead.

In my opinion, skin care products and prescription medications like retinoids do a better job of addressing your type's skin problems than facials. Plus, they are less expensive and less time-consuming. Retinoids will also help prevent wrinkles, another problem for your type, so see your dermatologist for a prescription.

## THE DOWNSIDE OF EASY SKIN

Having "easy" skin has certain disadvantages. To address a variety of skin problems from youth, other types used skin care products, which you never bothered with. These same products may have also conferred antiaging benefits, which you never received.

For example, in your teens, twenties, and thirties, while many of your peers agonized over acne, you had only occasional pimples. As a result, you never used a product like Retin-A, which in addition to lessening acne also has potent antiaging effects. Where many people with oily sensitive skin covered blemishes with foundation and powder, you never bothered with them, and missed out on the sun protection they provide. Because your skin is oily, you rarely used moisturizers and so you never got the extras they often contain, such as antioxidants, retinols, sunscreens, or other antiaging ingredients. ORNWs with dark skin never had to consult a dermatologist for help with dark spots, and therefore missed out on antiaging preparations.

Light-skinned ORNWs produce less melanin, a pigment that protects from sun damage. Without either pigmentation or sun protection, your skin is more exposed to harmful rays, and more at risk.

## AGING AND ORNW SKIN

Due to all these factors, in your thirties and beyond, many ORNWs are trying to play catch-up. Aging creeps up and catches you unaware. You may notice fine lines beginning to form on your forehead or between your eyebrows. Your jawline or neck begins to sag. Lines etch themselves at the corners of your mouth. While I'll offer skin care and treatment options to address these problems, if you're in your twenties or younger, be forewarned. Start protecting your skin *now.*

## A CLOSE-UP LOOK AT YOUR SKIN

With ORNW skin you may experience any of the following:

- Occasional bouts of facial shininess
- Minimal acne
- History of significant sun exposure in many cases
- No problem with most skin care products
- Difficulty tanning
- Little need to moisturize
- Early signs of wrinkles

## HOW WRINKLES FORM

Although wrinkles seem to appear overnight, that's not what really happens. Wrinkle formation occurs in stages. First, typically in your twenties, you will develop temporary "wrinkles in motion" in areas of facial movement such as around your eyes. These disappear when the corresponding muscle is relaxed. Later, often in your thirties, you will develop "wrinkles at rest" that remain visible even when the corresponding muscle is relaxed. Don't ignore the warning signs of first-stage wrinkles. The earlier they appear, the greater your tendency for deepening wrinkles over a lifetime. That's why wrinkle prevention is a must for your type.

The good news is that your skin's resilience and oiliness will permit you to tolerate the many treatments I'll recommend. But first and foremost, you must eliminate the ongoing sun exposure that damages skin and accelerates wrinkling.

## SELF-TANNERS

All self-tanners, including creams, lotions, gels, sprays, or the types they hose you down with at "fantasy tan" salons, contain the same active ingredient. It's called dihydroxyacetone (DHA), a sugar that interacts with amino acids in the upper layer of skin. The browning reaction that produces the "tan" is the same as when sugar-containing foods, like apples, turn brown after they are cut open and left to oxidize. Most self-tanners on the market contain 3–5 percent DHA. Because the upper skin layer is thicker over the elbows, knees, and palms, DHA-containing products cause more browning in these areas, so apply less self-tanner there.

To develop an even tan with these products, always use an exfoliating cream prior to application. Self-tanners provide no appreciable protection from the sun, with an SPF of only 1 or 2, which only lasts for an hour or two following application. Therefore, you should always use sunscreen as well.

Several sunless tanning products also contain antioxidants to ward off sun damage. Studies have shown that when self-tanners contain antioxidants, the end result is a more natural, less orange color. That's why I recommend that you seek out products such as Murad Self Tanner SPF 15.

## INDOOR TANNING

Indoor tanning was originally marketed as the "safe way to tan." Does that claim hold up? Not in my opinion. Tanning beds use ultraviolet A (UVA) rays to tan the skin. Since UVA does not cause an immediate skin reddening or sunburn as do UVB rays, people are not aware of the resulting long-term skin damage. UVA rays are more harmful than UVB because they penetrate more deeply into the dermis, the deeper layer of the skin, causing damage to collagen and other important skin proteins. The beautiful tan you see today can lead to premature aging, dark spots, and skin cancer tomorrow—or decades from now. If you are visiting a tanning bed, please stop. You are causing irreparable harm to your skin.

## SUNLESS TANNING BOOTHS

Sunless tanning booths were first introduced in 1999. These booths employ mobile or stationary misters that move 360 degrees around you to apply uniform amounts of sunless tanning solution to all parts of your body. While this assures a smooth product application that results in an even tan, tanning booth's spray-on self-tanners do have some downsides.

A recent FDA advisory cautioned against unwanted exposures to DHA, which may occur in sunless tanning booths. When eyes, lips, and mucous membranes are sprayed with DHA, some of the DHA may be ingested. The FDA advised people to cover and protect sensitive skin areas from receiving the spray, and from inadvertent ingestion or inhalation of DHA-containing products. Who is responsible for making sure you are protected if you go to a sunless tanning booth? Whatever the law may say, *you* are. Obviously, inhalation does not occur when you apply a cream or lotion tanner at home.

## WHAT CAN I DO TO PREVENT WRINKLES?

There are other ways to slow down your type's tendency to wrinkle. One key strategy is assuring that you get antioxidants, which combat free radicals and prevent aging. They can be ingested from foods, particularly fruits and vegetables, but I have found that when undertaking diets like the Atkins or South Beach, many people reduce their consumption of fruit. If your diet lacks ample fruits and vegetables, you can also obtain antioxidants from supplements. In addition, please check later in this chapter for my lists of antioxidant ingredients found in skin care products, as well as my recommendations for products containing these ingredients, well suited to your oily skin. Also consult pages 23 and 24 to find out more about factors contributing to skin aging. Beyond preventing wrinkles, you need to treat existing wrinkles, and I'll offer a range of suggestions to accomplish that.

## YOUR TREATMENT OPTIONS

Botulinum toxins like Botox inhibit muscle movement where wrinkles form, such as the crow's-feet around the eyes and frown lines, and may prevent the formation of future wrinkles as well. I personally hope it's true since I use them myself.

ORNWs can also use retinoids, prescription medications that help control oiliness and prevent wrinkles. While one particular brand, called Avage (which comes as a cream), is too strong for many types, you can easily tolerate it. In addition, because you don't develop dark spots after trauma and inflammation, you can also tolerate more aggressive wrinkle treatments such as laser resurfacing, dermabrasion, and deep chemical peels that other, more pigmented types must rule out. I'll recommend ones you can benefit from in the section on procedures later in this chapter.

Newly advanced wrinkle treatments beyond Botox that are currently in development will also be suitable for ORNWs. Currently, many dermal fillers, used to fill in wrinkles, are getting FDA approval. Restylane and Juvéderm are approved as treatments for facial wrinkles. As more fillers and botulinum toxins become available, increasing competition among suppliers will cause prices to come down, making these procedures more affordable.

People with wrinkled skin frequently wonder about a host of newly available and pricey creams advertised as "better than Botox." Although it seems appealing to get the same benefit out of a jar, I haven't seen any visible results from these creams beyond hydration, which any skin cream provides. Some of these creams use natural substances called peptides to make the top layer of the skin feel smoother. Their effect is like spackling a wall, which smoothes the surface but does not permanently change it.

My recommendation is that you save money for what you really need: prescription retinoids; botulinum toxins such as Botox or Dysport; and dermal fillers such as Restylane, Juvéderm, and Perlane.

If you're in your twenties or younger, don't take your skin for granted. Stop age-promoting habits such as smoking and sunbathing now. Take antioxidant supplements and use sunscreen and nonprescription retinol products or prescription retinoids to prevent aging. If you are thirty or older, you probably are beginning to have wrinkles. Using Botox or Dysport can prevent the wrinkles from worsening by preventing movement of the muscles in wrinkle-prone areas. Wearing sunglasses to prevent squinting will also help minimize the formation of eye wrinkles.

**Dr. Baumann's Bottom Line:** Splurge on the strong wrinkle treatments. Your skin can take it! After you repair the damage, turn your attention to prevention.

# EVERYDAY CARE FOR YOUR SKIN

The goal of your skin care routine is to address wrinkles and excess oil with wrinkle- and oil-control products that deliver antioxidants and retinols.

Many of you will want to see a dermatologist to have one of the many new wrinkle treatments that are available: lasers, dermabrasion, chemical peels, dermal fillers, or other procedures.

This regimen also includes products containing retinol and antioxidants that may help decrease your skin cancer risk.

## DAILY SKIN CARE

---

### REGIMEN

| AM | PM |
|---|---|
| Step 1: Wash with antioxidant cleanser | Step 1: Wash with same cleanser as in AM |
| Step 2: Apply toner, gel, or serum with antioxidants | Step 2: Use a facial scrub |
| Step 3: Apply sunscreen | Step 3: Apply a retinol- or retinaldehyde-containing product |
| Step 4: Apply oil-free foundation if you choose to wear it | |

---

In the morning, wash your face with a cleanser containing antioxidants to help prevent wrinkles. Then apply a toner, gel, or serum containing antioxidants. If your O/D score is very high (over 35), use a toner. If your score is lower (upper 20s or below), pick a serum or gel.

With a high O/D score (over 35), you should next use a mixture of an oil control gel and a gel sunscreen.

If your O/D score is between 24 and 34, instead of an oil control gel, apply a lotion sunscreen that contains antioxidants. Finally, apply an oil-free foundation if you would like to wear one.

In the evening, wash your face with the same cleanser you used in the morning, then use a facial scrub. Next, apply a product containing retinol or retinaldehyde. If you choose to use an eye cream, which is not necessary for your type, you can apply after cleansing.

You can remain on this regimen indefinitely. These OTC products are as good for your type as any prescription products—with the exception of the retinol/retinaldehyde product. I suggest instead that you see a dermatologist and get a prescription retinoid such as Avage, because the prescription product is stronger.

## Cleansers

ORNWs benefit from cleansers containing antioxidants, to help avoid wrinkles.

### RECOMMENDED CLEANSERS

- $ Clean & Clear Morning Burst Facial Cleanser with Bursting Beads
- $ Olay Total Effects Anti-Blemish Daily Cleanser
- $ Derma E Very Clear Problem Skin Cleanser
- $$ La Roche-Posay BioMedic Purifying Cleanser
- $$ Korres Thyme and Sage Facial Gel Cleanser
- $$ Mary Kay TimeWise 3-in-1 Cleanser
- $$ Peter Thomas Roth Anti-Aging Cleansing Gel
- $$ Philosophy Purity Made Simple One-Step Facial Cleanser
- $$ Topix Replenix Purifying Antioxidant Foaming Cleanser
- $$$ Elizabeth Arden Intervene Daily Cleanser
- $$$ Susan Ciminelli Cleansing Gel

**Baumann's Choice:** Topix Replenix Purifying Antioxidant Foaming Cleanser because it has antioxidants in it

## Toner Use

Toners are a great oil-free way to give your skin the antioxidants it needs. You can also use a gel or serum with oil-control properties and/or antioxidants.

One very beneficial antioxidant is green tea. Its proven benefits include protection from skin cancer and wrinkle prevention. You'll want to choose a product like Replenix serum, which contains such a high level of green tea that it is brown in color. But don't let the color put you off; if it isn't brown it simply doesn't have enough green tea for your purposes.

### RECOMMENDED TONERS, GELS, AND SERUMS

$ Olay Regenerist Daily Regenerating Serum
$$ Kiss My Face Potent and Pure C The Change, Ester C Serum
$$ SkinCeuticals Serum 20 (with ferulic acid)
$$ Topix CRS Cell Rejuvenation Serum
$$ Topix Replenix Retinol Smoothing Serum with green tea
$$$ Caudalie Vinopure Matte Finish Fluid
$$$ Elizabeth Arden Prevage Anti-Aging Treatment
$$$ Obagi Professional - C Serum 20%

**Baumann's Choice:** Replenix Retinol Smoothing Serum with green tea by Topix

## Oil Control

Toners don't control oil because they don't remain on the skin. Instead use an oil-control powder (recommendations appear later in this chapter) or an oil-control product with oil-absorbing ingredients, like these.

### RECOMMENDED OIL-CONTROL PRODUCTS

$$ OC Eight Professional Mattifying Gel
$$ Mary Kay Oil Mattifier
$$ Paula's Choice Skin Balancing Super Antioxidant Mattifying Concentrate
$$$ Smashbox Anti-Shine Powder-Gel

**Baumann's Choice:** Paula's Choice Skin Balancing Super Antioxidant Mattifying Concentrate because it has retinol, oil control, and antioxidants

## Moisturizers

You don't need a morning moisturizer. Use one of the recommended serums instead. You may need an evening moisturizer if you have a lower O/D score (below 35).

## RECOMMENDED MOISTURIZERS

- $    Alpha Hydrox Oil-Free Formula
- $    Neutrogena Visibly Firm Night Cream
- $    Mario Badescu Control Moisturizer for Oily Skin
- $$   Mary Kay TimeWise Age-Fighting Moisturizer
- $$   Replenix CF Cream by Topix
- $$$  SkinCeuticals Renew Overnight Oily

**Baumann's Choice:** Replenix CF Cream because it contains a high amount of green tea, a powerful antioxidant. They are coming out with a new one soon with Resveratrol called the Power of Three cream, so watch for that one.

## Eye Creams

Eye creams are not necessary, but if you choose to use one, select a product with antiaging ingredients.

## RECOMMENDED EYE CREAMS

- $    Aveeno Ageless Vitality Elasticity Recharging System-Eye
- $    Skin Effects Eye Effects Dual Action Under Eye Therapy
- $$   Cellex-C Eye Contour Gel
- $$   MD Skincare Lift & Lighten Eye Cream
- $$   SkinCeuticals Eye Gel
- $$$  Dr. Brandt Lineless Eye Cream
- $$$  Elizabeth Arden Prevage Anti-Aging Eye Treatment
- $$$  Relastin Eye Silk

**Baumann's Choice:** Aveeno Ageless Vitality Elasticity Recharging System-Eye. The copper- and zinc-containing cream creates a charge that stimulates cells to make elastin. It is followed by a cream with blackberry and dill extract that also help increase the skin's elasticity.

## Wrinkle Prevention

The only effective nonprescription topical products for preventing wrinkles contain retinols or antioxidants, but their efficacy depends on the concentration offered in the product. The ones I recommend here are good options.

## RECOMMENDED WRINKLE-
## PREVENTION PRODUCTS

$ Neutrogena Healthy Skin Anti-Wrinkle Cream
$ RoC Retinol Correxion Deep Wrinkle Night Cream
$$ Replenix Retinol Smoothing Serum 5X
$$ La Roche-Posay Active C Normal/Combination Skin
$$ Philosophy Help Me (retinol treatment)
$$ Kinerase Lotion with Kinetin & Zeatin
$$$ Elizabeth Arden Prevage

**Baumann's Choice:** Replenix Retinol Smoothing Serum 5X or Philosophy's Help Me are very similar; choose whichever is easiest to find and/or cheapest.

## Exfoliation

For ORNWs, an at-home exfoliating scrub or microdermabrasion kit will provide the same results as a spa or salon microdermabrasion treatment.

## RECOMMENDED EXFOLIATION PRODUCTS

$ Boots No7 Total Renewal Micro-Dermabrasion Exfoliator
$ Specific Beauty Exfoliating Cleansing Cloths
$ Olay Regenerist Microdermabrasion & Peel System
$ Skin Effects Purifying Effects Deep-Cleansing Enzyme Scrub
$$ Philosophy Never Let Them See You Shine Scrub
$$ Vivite Exfoliating Cleanser
$$$ The Clarisonic MD Professional Skin Care Brush

**Baumann's Choice:** Vivite Exfoliating Cleanser because I love the texture and the fact that it has glycolic acid. I also have to admit that I think the packaging of the entire Vivite line is beautiful.

## SHOPPING FOR PRODUCTS

You can widen your choice of products by reading labels to determine product ingredients; thus, you can select those that contain beneficial ingredients for avoiding wrinkles, while steering clear of ingredients that cause oiliness.

If you find favorite products that are not listed in your chapter, please go to www.skintypesolutions.com and share your finds with me.

## SKIN CARE INGREDIENTS TO USE

### *To prevent wrinkles:*

- Caffeine
- Coenzyme $Q_{10}$ (ubiquinone)
- Copper peptide
- Ginseng
- Grape seed extract
- Green tea
- *Humulus lupulus* (hops)
- Idebenone
- Lutein
- Lycopene
- Moringa
- *Pinus pinaster* (pine bark)
- Pomegranate
- Resveratrol
- Rosemary
- Vitamin C (ascorbic acid)
- Vitamin E

### *To treat wrinkles:*

- Alpha lipoic acid
- Copper peptide
- DMAE
- Glycolic acid (AHA)
- Lactic acid (AHA)
- Phytic acid (AHA)
- Retinol
- Salicylic acid (BHA)
- TGF-Beta
- Vitamin C (ascorbic acid)

## SKIN CARE INGREDIENTS TO AVOID

### *Due to excess oiliness:*

- Mineral oil
- Other oils such as safflower oil
- Petrolatum

## Sun Protection for Your Skin

Using a sunscreen is especially important for ORNWs. If you have a high O/D score (above 35), you will want to use facial powders with sunscreen. Whether you like to use several different makeup products, such as powder, foundation, and primer, or whether you prefer to simply wear a single product, like sunscreen, make sure you reach the minimum SPF of 15, which I advise for daily use. If your O/D score is between 30 and 34, choose a gel sunscreen. Those with O/D scores lower than 30 may prefer lotion sunscreens.

If you prefer not to use a facial foundation or powder with SPF, use one of the sunscreens listed later in this section.

## When and How to Apply Sunscreen

Apply sunscreen every morning, even if you don't expect to go outdoors. Staying indoors will not protect you. UVA easily penetrates windows to send harmful sun rays into buildings, cars, and airplanes. Keep sunscreen in your car, desk, and purse to reapply if needed. Please find detailed instructions for sunscreen application on pages 21 and 22.

### RECOMMENDED SUN PROTECTION PRODUCTS

- $ Neutrogena Ultra Sheer Dry-Touch Sunblock with Helioplex
- $$ La Roche-Posay Anthelios 60 Ultra Light Sunscreen Fluid Extreme, SPF 60
- $$ SkinCeuticals Daily Sun Defense SPF 20
- $$$ Clarins Oil-Free Sun Care Spray SPF 15

**Baumann's Choice:** La Roche-Posay Anthelios 60 Ultra Light Sunscreen Fluid Extreme, SPF 60 containing Mexoryl and several other sun-blocking ingredients, or Neutrogena Ultra Sheer Dry-Touch Sunblock with Helioplex

## Your Makeup

Avoid oil-containing foundations and instead use powders that absorb oil. Many foundations are marked "oil free" on the label, but some that claim to control oiliness actually contain oil. To find out whether yours does, get a piece of 25 percent–cotton bond paper. Place a drop of foundation on it.

Oil-containing foundations will leave a ring of oil on the paper. The size of the ring is proportional to the amount of oil in the foundation—the bigger the ring, the more oil the product contains.

### RECOMMENDED OIL-FREE FOUNDATIONS

- $ Avon MagiX Tinted Face Perfector
- $$ Bobbi Brown Oil-Free Even Finish Foundation SPF 15
- $$ Flawless Finish Bare Perfection Makeup SPF 8
- $$ Laura Mercier Oil-Free Foundation
- $$ Stila Natural Finish Oil Free Makeup

**Baumann's Choice:** I prefer those with SPF.

### RECOMMENDED OIL-ABSORBING POWDERS

- $ CoverGirl Clean Pressed Powder
- $ Maybelline Shine Free Oil-Control Pressed Powder
- $ Revlon ColorStay Pressed Powder
- $$ Bobbi Brown Sheer Finish Loose Powder
- $$ Jane Iredale "PurePressed" Base SPF 20
- $$$ Chanel Pureté Mat Shine Control Powder SPF 15
- $$$ Laura Mercier Foundation Powder

**Baumann's Choice:** Jane Iredale "PurePressed" Base SPF 20

## PROCEDURES FOR YOUR SKIN TYPE

Skin care procedures for this type concentrate on treating wrinkles. Follow my skin care recommendations to prevent wrinkles, but to address wrinkles that have already formed, you may want to indulge in the procedures I recommend below to get rid of them.

## PROCEDURES TO TREAT WRINKLES

You have a choice of a range of procedures for treating wrinkles. They include injections of botulinum toxin, like Botox, dermal fillers, or dermabrasion.

# Dermabrasion

While the advanced procedures will help with many kinds of wrinkles, stubborn wrinkles around the mouth, called "smoker's lines," are hard to treat permanently. People with lighter skin (which includes the majority of ORNWs), have an additional option in dermabrasion (which is not to be confused with microdermabrasion).

In the dermabrasion procedure, the physician uses a tiny spinning wheel covered with diamonds to remove the top layer of skin down to the depth of the dermis (the deeper of the two main layers that make up the skin). This level of skin removal is much deeper than occurs in microdermabrasion, which uses tiny crystals that gently abrade the skin, removing only the upper layer of dead skin cells.

Be prepared to take some time off following dermabrasion, since afterward the treated skin will have an open sore for about four to seven days. Once that heals, you may experience anywhere from a few days to a few weeks of redness. Fortunately, that can be covered by makeup.

The good news is that when the skin heals, it appears much smoother and less lined. However, this procedure does carry some risks, including scarring and lightening of the skin in the treated area. That is why I do not advise this option unless you go to a highly qualified doctor who is experienced in performing the procedure. Admittedly, not many are available. Please consult the Resources section for information on how to find a qualified dermatologist.

Unlike people with pigmented skin, light-skinned ORNWs are good candidates for dermabrasion because they do not develop dark spots in the treated areas. (Someone with tight skin would not require dermabrasion since wrinkles are not an issue.)

Although this procedure may sound scary, I have been amazed by the lack of pain that people report and the results achieved. You may have heard about $CO_2$ laser resurfacing, which previously was used to get rid of these stubborn lines around the mouth. It has fallen out of favor because many patients reported long-term complications. Dermabrasion has been safely performed for over thirty-five years.

# Microdermabrasion

Microdermabrasion, a popular procedure offered in dermatology offices, skin care salons, and spas, removes the upper dead layer of skin to make your skin feel smoother. The practitioner uses a device that sprays microcrystals to remove the upper surface layer of the skin. As an ORNW, you can freely benefit from microdermabrasion treatments, although frankly, an exfoliating scrub or microdermabrasion home kit will provide the same results, for less cost. (Save the money for what you really need: prescription retinoids and dermal fillers.) Nevertheless, if you want to look radiant for a party, and you have the time and the money—go for it. Or else, try something disposable, like the Specific Beauty Exfoliating Cleansing Cloths. See the list of exfoliators and microdermabrasion at-home kits for more suggestions.

## Lasers

A new technique called Ulthera can treat droopy lines around the mouth and nose area as well as the under-neck sagging skin, which gives a "turkey neck" appearance.

## Spa Procedures

ORNWs are great candidates for spa and cosmetic dermatology services like chemical peels, which help exfoliate skin.

Microcurrent units popular in many facial salons are electrical devices that stimulate the facial muscles to contract or stretch, aiming to relax tight muscles and tone loose ones; but it isn't clear whether this treatment is effective, since the appearance of aging is mostly caused by loss of fat as we age, which causes the skin to lose volume.

As an ORNW considering salon services, be warned: Salon services may not be powerful enough for you. Your resistant skin can handle high-strength chemical peels, which are usually not performed in spas, so make sure to ask for a higher concentration than they use on their sensitive-skin clients.

## What About Lights?

Light treatments such as light-emitting diodes and Intense Pulsed Light will probably become important in the future to prevent or treat wrinkles. At this time, the technology is still being improved as far as wrinkles are concerned. I am dismayed by the number of patients I see who have already spent $5,000 to $6,000 on these treatments and have not seen any difference in their wrinkles. (These treatments are great for removing blood vessels, redness, and dark spots, which are not concerns for ORNWs.)

## Ongoing Care for Your Skin

Focus on wrinkle prevention. If it's too late, don't be afraid to bite the bullet and do something that really works! Your RN skin helps protect you from the side effects that other Skin Types develop after more intensive procedures.

# CHAPTER ELEVEN

# Oily, Resistant, Non-Pigmented, and Tight: ORNT

## BAUMANN SKIN TYPE NUMBER 10

■

*"My main concern is oiliness. Do I need a moisturizer? How do I find a sunscreen that does not make me shiny? What tips do you have to reduce that midday shine?"*

### ABOUT YOUR SKIN

Flawless, even toned, radiant, ageless.

If you're an ORNT, you won the Skin Type lottery—although you probably never knew there was one. You rarely think about your skin. It's easy to care for, plus it always looks great. You don't understand all the fuss about skin care. You wouldn't dream of springing big bucks for procedures or surgery.

Frankly, if you're an ORNT, I'm surprised and flattered that you bought this book. Why? Because you have one of the easiest Skin Types to care for, age in, and live with overall. In you, lucky genes and good skin care habits combine to create age-defying skin. Your oily, tight skin protects you from the visible signs of aging while your skin cells produce color without any tendency to develop dark spots after trauma or inflammation. If you have a light skin tone, you may have some trouble tanning, but so what? Having youthful skin throughout your life is a good trade-off for the temporary thrill of a tan, especially when you consider that tanning promotes aging. Unlike Sensitive or Dry Skin Types, ORNTs do not get acne, redness, dark spots, or dryness.

## YOUR SKIN HISTORY

In youth, your skin probably tended to be oily, but as you reach your forties, you'll find that your skin begins to normalize and becomes less so. While other forty-year-olds fight dryness, your skin is just right. Some of you are so proud of your skin that you pamper it with various creams and concoctions, avoiding sunning and smoking to preserve your skin's beauty. Others with this type do everything wrong: you smoke, sunbathe, go without adequate sleep, and use whatever soap happens to be lying around, without a thought. In that case, your skin seems to exemplify the power of genetics.

ORNTs with darker skin tones are free of the cycle of acne and dark spots that troubles many people of color. Though an occasional cut or trauma, like a burn, scrape, or irritation, could lead to a temporary dark spot, this occurs so infrequently that there's little need to prevent it in your Daily Skin Care Regimen. Dark-skinned ORNTs may develop dark spots and temporarily become pigmented types due to the hormonal shifts that occur during pregnancy. However, don't worry, as your skin will return to its native N, or non-pigmented state, soon after your hormones return to postpregnancy levels. Lighter-skinned ORNTs are not prone to hormonally related pigmentation experienced by people of color.

## A CLOSE-UP LOOK AT YOUR SKIN

With ORNT skin you may experience any of the following:

- Smooth, oily skin
- Little need for moisturizer
- Few wrinkles
- Foundation makeup streaks
- Large pores
- Blackheads
- Enlarged oil glands
- Infrequent acne breakouts
- Skin cancers (see next page so that you can identify the signs)

Genes determine how much pigment (melanin) your skin produces. Most non-pigmented types produce less than pigmented types, while a light-skinned, non-pigmented type will have even less than a dark-skinned ORNT. Increased melanin lowers your risk of skin cancer. With less skin pigment, there is less protection against the deleterious effects of the sun. As a result, light-skinned ORNTs are more vulnerable to skin cancer than dark-skinned ORNTs. Check yourself, and double-check with a dermatologist regularly.

## How to Recognize a Non-Melanoma Skin Cancer

A squamous cell carcinoma (SCC) may appear as red, scaling patches that form scabs in sun-exposed areas such as the face, ears, chest, arms, legs, and back. They do not heal. They may be covered by a hard white scale that resembles a wart. Any spot that fits this description and persists for one month or more should be seen by a dermatologist.

A basal cell carcinoma (BCC) may appear as a white, shiny bump, luminous like a pearl. They may have either a central ridge with a little hole or depression, or tiny blood vessels visible in the border. They can also look like a crater or scar that suddenly appears although there has been no prior trauma. Sometimes the border is "ruffled" or heaped up around the central crater.

Enlarged facial oil glands can be easily confused with BCC, since they both are yellowish bumps. Make sure to check out anything suspicious with a dermatologist. Your skin cancer risk is one of this type's only downsides. Take it seriously, and get regular checkups.

## HOW GENES OPERATE IN SKIN AGING

Genes regulate the production of collagen and elastin, the key skin proteins responsible for skin firmness and resilience. Many skin care products contain these ingredients, claiming to deliver them topically. But without studies documenting these claims, I don't find their promises convincing. Cosmetic companies have also tried to capitalize on the emerging science of aging by customizing skin care products based on genetic testing. However, we don't yet know how to use that information to create an effective product. Perhaps we will in ten or twenty years, but right now, in my opinion, the promise of individualized genetic-based treatments is just clever marketing and beautiful packaging to sell the same old stuff at higher prices. Until we know how to replicate the genetic factors that make skin great, invest in your future by adopting the positive lifestyle factors that we do know can help.

Most people wonder, "How gracefully will I age?" While neither I nor this book's questionnaire can predict that absolutely, a few simple certainties and some other subtle tendencies can reveal how well you'll age and what you can and *should* do to maintain youthful skin.

For people with tight, unwrinkled skin, genetics play a key role. Confirming this, you will probably notice that your mother, grandmother, or other relatives aged gracefully and looked younger than their contemporaries even in advanced years.

I commonly hear from my ORNT patients statements like, "I take after my mother's side of the family. Both my mother and grandmother had great skin," or, "My grandmother told people she was sixty when she was really seventy-five and everyone believed her!"

Build on this good foundation with skin-enhancing lifestyle habits like avoiding sun exposure. Don't weaken that foundation with poor ones, like tanning, smoking, or going to tanning beds. Even those with good genes can wind up with more wrinkles if they indulge in the latter habits. I've seen pictures of identical twins, one with sun exposure, one without, and the one without looked much younger.

Have empathy for the other types since your Skin Type is uncommon. Don't expect your children, guests, or spouses to be able to use skin care products as indiscriminately as you can. One application of that same nicely scented hotel lotion that you use without a second thought, and I, for one, develop red and itching skin for twenty-four hours.

How to take the best care of your skin? Unless you are troubled by oiliness, you don't need to do anything special, other than remembering to apply sunscreen. Overall, my product recommendations will be kinder to your skin than that deodorant soap you happen to use. While maintaining ORNT skin is not hard work, why not treat your skin right with appropriate skin care?

## YOUR MOST BASIC SKIN CARE STRATEGIES

If you have excessive oil, use the oil-control products I'll recommend. If you are prone to blackheads, prevent them with prescription retinoids. Use powders instead of makeup foundations when possible. Don't be tricked into wasting money on toners, serums, or antiaging night creams, because you don't need them.

Since you have easy, resistant skin, feel free to experiment. You can tolerate fragrant skin creams, all types of ingredients, and preservatives. Getting facials is probably a great treat for you, even when the aesthetician uses products that can irritate many of us. Enjoy, count your blessings, and feel free to add variety to your skin care routine.

Your recommendations include products that are more adventurous than those I suggest to other types. If you develop a problem, recheck your questionnaire responses. You may be an OSNT who in the past has used less adventurous products so that you did not realize that your skin is sensitive. Changing environments, increased stress, or changes in lifestyle habits can also cause your Skin Type to change.

**Dr. Baumann's Bottom Line:** Whatever combination of good genes and good skin care gave you your youthful line-free skin, help out nature and prevent skin cancer through good skin care and avoiding excess sun exposure.

## EVERYDAY CARE FOR YOUR SKIN

Your skin care routine focuses on addressing skin oiliness with products that deliver oil-absorbing ingredients or contain ingredients that will to a certain extent decrease oil production. Unfortunately, not many products are able to permanently and totally decrease your skin's production of oil. This makes ongoing control essential. Your daily regimen will also treat and prevent pore enlargement, treat and prevent blackheads, and prevent occasional acne breakouts.

First, look over the regimen and then you can choose the products you'll need from those I recommend in each category later in this chapter.

If after using this regimen for two months, you still have trouble with occasional acne, you may wish to consult a dermatologist, who can prescribe retinoids.

Since ORNT is the easiest Skin Type to care for, I've built a one-stage regimen geared toward decreasing oil production to help treat and prevent your infrequent acne breakouts as well as minimizing enlarged pores. The products you'll use will soak up excess oil and decrease facial shine.

## DAILY SKIN CARE

### REGIMEN

| AM | PM |
|---|---|
| Step 1: Wash with cleanser | Step 1: Wash with cleanser |
| Step 2: Apply oil-control product | Step 2: Use a scrub or exfoliator (optional) |
| Step 3: Apply oil-free foundation with oil control (optional) | Step 3: Apply a retinol product |
| Step 4: Apply powder with SPF | |

In the morning, wash your face with one of the recommended cleansers. Apply an oil-control product. If you have a higher O/D score (above 35), you may wish to wear oil-free foundation and/or makeup powder with SPF as well. Remember: Make sure to wear at least one product that contains SPF 15. Everyone needs sun protection. You may also wish to carry blotting papers with you to absorb oil, whenever needed.

In the evening, wash with cleanser, and then you can use a scrub two to three times per week. Next, use a retinol-containing product to help lessen oil production.

## Cleansers

To control your skin's oil production, keep your skin clean. Excess oil clogs pores and stretches them out, resulting in enlarged pores. Products that claim to shrink pores really just irritate the skin, causing the pores to swell so that they look smaller temporarily. Nothing can permanently shrink pores, but products containing beta hydroxy acid (BHA) can penetrate into pores and clear them, thereby minimizing pore enlargement. Be sure to use cleanser both morning and evening.

### RECOMMENDED CLEANSING PRODUCTS

$ Aveeno Clear Complexion Foaming Cleanser
$ Neutrogena Oil-Free Acne Wash Pink Grapefruit Facial Cleanser

$   Cetaphil Daily Facial Cleanser for Normal to Oily Skin
$$  Topix Gly Sal 5-2 Cleanser
$$  Wai Hope Sea Rescue Purifying Cleanser
$$  Peter Thomas Roth Glycolic Acid 3% Facial Wash
$$  Philosophy Purity Made Simple One-step Facial Cleanser

**Baumann's Choice:** Wai Hope Sea Rescue Purifying Cleanser because it contains organic ingredients

## Toner Use

Some oily types enjoy the refreshing, clean feeling that toners provide. Although they will not control oil as well as the oil-control cleansers, foundations, and powder, if you'd like to use a toner, feel free to do so. It will not harm your skin, though in my opinion it's an unnecessary expense. If you do use a toner, you might try any of these I recommend.

### RECOMMENDED TONERS

$  Neutrogena Pore Refining Toner, Alpha and Beta Hydroxy Formula
$  Burt's Bees Garden Tomato Toner for Oily and Troubled Skin
$  Boots Botanics Skin Brightening Toner
$$  Dr. Hauschka Clarifying Toner (for oily skin)
$$  Kiehl's Rare Earth Pore Refining Tonic
$$  Murad Clarifying Toner
$$  PCA Skin Nutrient Toner
$$  Paula's Choice Skin Balancing Toner
$$$  Chanel Precision Lotion Confort Silky Soothing Toner Comfort + Anti-Pollution
$$$  Darphin Niaouli Aromatic Care Toner
$$$  Natura Bisse Stabilizing Toner

**Baumann's Choice:** Burt's Bees Garden Tomato Toner for Oily and Troubled Skin

## Oil-Control Products

Retinol products may also help to decrease oiliness and prevent outbreaks. Applying oil-free makeup foundations, foundation primers, and powders will absorb oil and reduce the appearance of oiliness. Since no ingredients can totally control oil secretion, stay on top of your skin's native oiliness by blotting with the products recommended below. You can address blackheads, when they occur, with Bioré Deep Cleansing Pore Strips.

## RECOMMENDED OIL-CONTROL PRODUCTS

$ Seban liquid
$ Seban pads
$$ Jack Black All Day Oil-Control Lotion
$$ OC Eight Professional Mattifying Gel
$$$ Dr. Brandt Pores No More Pore Refiner

**Baumann's Choice:** Dr. Brandt Pores No More Pore Refiner

## RETINOL-CONTAINING PRODUCTS

$ Neutrogena Ageless Intensives Deep Wrinkle Anti-Wrinkle Serum
$ RoC Retinol Correxion Deep Wrinkle Night Cream
$$ Afirm 2x or Afirm 3x
$$ Philosophy Help Me (retinol treatment)
$$ Replenix Retinol Plus Smoothing Serum 5x

**Baumann's Choice:** Replenix Retinol Plus Smoothing Serum 5x with a high amount of retinol, packaged properly to ensure stability of retinol

## RECOMMENDED BLOTTERS

$ Clean & Clear Oil Absorbing Sheets
$ Mary Kay Beauty Blotters Oil-Absorbing Tissues
$ Paula's Choice Oil Blotting Papers
$ The Body Shop Tea Tree Oil Facial Blotting Tissues

**Baumann's Choice:** Any of the above

## Moisturizers

With very oily skin, you generally will not need to moisturize. However, you may find that in drier climates and when the humidity is low, as in winter, your skin feels tight. If so, a light moisturizer can help. If you have a lower O/D score (27 to 35) you may have combination skin and require a moisturizer. If so, choose a light one from among those I suggest and apply it in drier skin areas. Finally, as you age, oiliness will decrease, so that using a light moisturizer becomes an option.

### RECOMMENDED MOISTURIZERS

$ Paula's Choice Skin Balancing Moisture Gel
$$ Clinique Dramatically Different Moisturizing Gel
$$ Topix Replenix CF Cream or Serum
$$$ ReVive Intensite Moisture Serum Extreme

**Baumann's Choice:** Topix Replenix CF Cream or Serum—the gel form keeps it from being too greasy.

## Masks

You can apply a mask to temporarily decrease skin oiliness. Use one prior to a party or at any time when you do not want your face to look shiny in photographs.

### RECOMMENDED MASKS

$ Boots Botanics Conditioning Clay Mask
$ Queen Helene Natural English Clay Mud Pack Masque
$$ Darphin Purifying Aromatic Clay Mask
$$ DDF Sulfur Therapeutic Mask
$$ Nars Mud Mask
$$$ Dr. Michelle Copeland Clay Mask

**Baumann's Choice:** Boots Botanics Conditioning Clay Mask because of the price, but they are all good

## Exfoliation

ORNTs can benefit from scrubs and microdermabrasion to help keep pores clean and trouble free.

## RECOMMENDED FACIAL SCRUBS

$   L'Oréal ReFinish Micro-Dermabrasion Kit

$   BeautiControl Spa Resurface Microderm Abrasion for Face

$$   Neutrogena Wave Power-Cleanser and Deep Clean Foaming Pads

$$   Bioré Pore Unclogging Scrub

$$   The Body Shop Seaweed Foaming Facial Scrub

$$   Philosophy Microdelivery Peel

$$$   Dr. Brandt Microdermabrasion in a Jar

$$$   Clarisonic Mia with GoClear Clarifying Cleanser

**Baumann's Choice:** L'Oréal ReFinish Micro-Dermabrasion Kit. It comes with a moisturizer that those of you with oilier skin may not need. Instead, it makes a fantastic hand cream.

## SHOPPING FOR PRODUCTS

There are no specific ingredients that you need to look for in skin care products. However, you should choose products labeled "oil control" and avoid those containing mineral oil and other oils such as sunflower oil and borage seed oil.

### SKIN CARE INGREDIENTS TO AVOID

*Due to excess oil:*

- Borage seed oil
- Mineral oil
- Other oils
- Petrolatum
- Sunflower oil

## Sun Protection for Your Skin

For your type, I prefer gels and sprays, I suggest you avoid cream sunscreen, because it tends to make skin feel and appear oilier. However, if you will be receiving prolonged sun exposure, you can use the gel sunscreens I recommend. For complete instructions on sunscreen use, please refer to Chapter Two.

## RECOMMENDED SUN PROTECTION PRODUCTS, POWDERS

$   Colorescience SPF 20

$   L'Oréal Air Wear Powder Foundation SPF 17

$$   Elizabeth Arden Flawless Finish Dual Perfection Makeup SPF 8

$$   Philosophy Supernatural Air Brushed Canvas

$$   Stila Sheer Color Face Powder SPF 15

$$   Vichy Capital Soleil

$$$   Bobbi Brown Sheer Finish Loose Powder

$$$   Shu Uemura UV Under Base SPF 8

**Baumann's Choice:** All are fine but do not depend on the sun protection in these products. You must use a separate sunscreen.

## RECOMMENDED SUN PROTECTION PRODUCTS, GELS, AND SPRAYS

$   Aveeno Continuous Protection Sunblock Lotion for the face SPF 30

$   Bull Frog Quik Gel Sport Spray Sunblock, SPF 36

$   Neutrogena Ultra Sheer Dry-Touch Sunblock with Helioplex

$$   La Roche-Posay Anthelios 60 Ultra Light Sunscreen Fluid Extreme, SPF 60

$$$   Clarins Oil-Free Sun Care Spray SPF 15

**Baumann's Choice:** La Roche-Posay Anthelios 60 Ultra Light Sunscreen Fluid Extreme, SPF 60, Neutrogena Ultra Sheer Dry-Touch Sunblock, or the Aveeno.

## Your Makeup

Here you can enjoy and experiment. Unlike some other types, you should not experience reactions to any colors or pigments typically found in makeup products, nor are there any types of makeup you need to avoid.

The powders and foundations I recommend help reduce shine by surrounding the oil, making it less visible on the skin, or else by absorbing the oil. Talc and kaolin in these products help absorb oil. Use oil-control powders to prevent the makeup streaking that often comes with very oily skin. If you have a lower O/D score, you can wear foundations without a problem.

If your score is high (above 35), either skip the foundation and use only a powder, or use an oil-absorbing foundation primer.

Foundation primers absorb oil when applied before a foundation and enable the foundation to last longer without streaking. You can also use them on their own, without foundation.

## RECOMMENDED FOUNDATION PRIMERS

- $ Boots No7 Mattifying Makeup Base
- $ The Body Shop Matte It Face & Lips
- $$ Elizabeth Arden Good Morning Skin Serum
- $$ Laura Mercier Foundation Primer
- $$$ Smashbox Photo Finish Foundation Primer Light
- $$$ Lancôme La Base Pro Perfecting Makeup Primer Smoothing Effect, Oil Free

**Baumann's Choice:** Laura Mercier Foundation Primer

## RECOMMENDED FOUNDATIONS

- $ Iman Second To None Oil-Free Makeup, SPF 8
- $ Neutrogena SkinClearing Foundation and Powder
- $$ Philosophy The Supernatural Airbrushed Canvas Powder Foundation
- $$ Stila Illuminating Powder Foundation

**Baumann's Choice:** Iman Second To None Oil-Free Makeup, SPF 8 has many colors good for darker-skinned people.

## RECOMMENDED OIL-CONTROL POWDERS

- $ Maybelline Shine Free Oil-Control Pressed Powder
- $$ Fashion Fair Oil-Control Loose Face Powder
- $$ Jurlique Rose Silk Powder
- $$ Prescriptives Virtual Matte Oil-Control Pressed Powder
- $$$ Estée Lauder Double Matte Oil-Control Pressed Powder
- $$$ Shu Uemura Face Powder Matte

**Baumann's Choice:** Fashion Fair Oil-Control Loose Face Powder

## PROCEDURES FOR YOUR SKIN TYPE

ORNTs don't need any procedures. Yes, that's right! If you look at the chapters for other Skin Types, you'll see that I don't hesitate to recommend advanced skin options when needed. But you really don't need them. So get yourself a new pair of shoes instead!

That being said, if you want to give yourself some extra pampering, there are a few options you can consider. For instance, you might try microdermabrasion to smooth and soften your skin. Women who have tried it report that their makeup goes on smoother, making pores just a little more refined.

However, I feel that the scrubs suggested earlier give the same result at a much lower cost and time commitment. Of course, you could always plump your lips with collagen or hyaluronic acid, but you probably do not need botulinum toxins, lasers, or chemical peels.

ORNTs are very lucky. If you make good lifestyle choices such as sun avoidance, smoking cessation, and consumption of a diet high in antioxidants, you should enjoy many years of good skin. Your skin's oiliness tends to decrease in your forties and fifties, so that, unlike other types, your skin actually gets better with time.

In your late fifties and sixties, you may begin to experience some skin dryness, but using a light moisturizer should be enough to correct this.

Hormone fluctuations can lead to skin oiliness as well. If you are female and this is a troublesome issue for you, you may want to consider an oral contraceptive. Ask your doctor which low-androgen product is right for you.

## ONGOING CARE FOR YOUR SKIN

Rejoice! You have the easiest Skin Type. But don't take your good luck for granted. Maintain good skin care habits, and regularly check to assure that new moles or growths are not skin cancers. Plus, keep eating those vegetables.

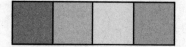

## PART FOUR

# Skin Care for Dry, Sensitive Skin

# CHAPTER TWELVE

# Dry, Sensitive, Pigmented, and Wrinkled: DSPW

## BAUMANN SKIN TYPE NUMBER 3

*"I have many issues with my skin, including aging. I am over-whelmed by the product choices out there. It seems as if I need to use too many different products on my skin. Can you help me streamline my regimen and identify an easy skin regimen that addresses my particular concerns?"*

## ABOUT YOUR SKIN

A DSPW Skin Type gives you no slack. Your skin is dry, flaky, parched, and crying out for moisturizers. Yet you react with pimples or stinging, burning, and itching to so many ingredients that few products can help. Synthetic ingredients in skin care (such as fragrances, detergents, and preservatives) can trigger a reaction. Natural ingredients in skin care (such as essential oils, coconut oil, or cocoa butter) can also trigger a reaction.

When using a product to treat your dark spots, it may sting and turn your pigmented skin red. Even though you avoid the sun, people frequently ask if you've been to the beach, because your red flushed face makes you look sunburned even in the dead of winter. Antiaging creams make you look like a burn victim, leaving inflamed red patches that turn brown over time and take months to heal.

Though improving your skin will be a careful step-by-step process, it can be done, so do not give up. The good news is that of all the types, DSPWs will gain the most from this book. Fortunately, there has been a great deal of research into your type that I'll translate into clear recommendations to help you improve your skin and with it your quality of life.

## THE DSPW DOUBLE BIND

Your skin's hyperreactivity is not your imagination. With one of the most distressing Skin Types, you find it difficult to care for properly. Though friends with easier types don't understand, I can validate your experience. Unless you're a millionaire who can afford to buy dozens of products, then use and discard them when they don't work, it's nearly impossible to find your way through the labyrinth of skin care products to the select few that work for your skin.

DSPWs often have eczema, also called atopic dermatitis, a skin condition in which dry skin becomes irritated, reddened, and inflamed before developing patches that itch and take awhile to heal. Please refer to pages 208 and 209 for a more detailed description of eczema and the factors exacerbating this condition. If allowed to persist, the condition is both physically uncomfortable and psychologically embarrassing, since it's visible to others.

## A DISTURBED SKIN BARRIER

Dry, sensitive types have a disturbed skin barrier. The cells that maintain the integrity of the skin have broken down as a result of different causes— including allergies, sensitizing products and ingredients, and environmental conditions, like dryness and cold. As a result, the barrier doesn't keep water in, so the skin lacks the hydration it needs. On the other hand, it also doesn't keep allergenic ingredients out. When these ingredients invade, they trigger inflammation.

DSPWs have no protection. You are literally thin-skinned. The resulting dryness, irritation, redness, and itchiness give you the urge to scratch, but scratching further attacks your skin barrier. Next, pigmentation causes skin darkening at irritated areas, such as the back of the knees and inside of the elbows. Scratches, cuts, and scrapes are more than uncomfortable: They can result in dark spots at the site of injury because your skin's high pigment levels react to any inflammation. It's a vicious cycle.

Dark spots can result from many causes, including cuts, scratches, oral contraceptive use, pregnancy, and sun exposure. The dark spots appear darker in the summer if the skin is tanned. Dark patches resulting from injury more commonly occur in dark-skinned people. Dermatologists call them post-inflammatory pigmentation alteration (PIPA). Both dark- and light-skin-toned DSPWs can suffer from melasma (also called "the mask of pregnancy"), which results from sun exposure and higher estrogen levels.

Eczema can occur anywhere on your body. To find out if you suffer from this problem, please go to "Do I Have Eczema?" in Chapter Thirteen. Skin dryness, redness, and irritation can appear on your face and neck, while scaling dry patches frequently crop up behind the ears. As if all this were not stressful enough, eczema *worsens* with stress. In more severe cases, sufferers may experience sleep problems due to discomfort. Given the frequency of flare-ups, sleep loss is more than occasional. One study revealed that those with a moderate form of eczema suffer flare-ups for three months a year, while severe patients may experience flare-ups for five months a year. Irritable, uncomfortable, embarrassed, and sleep-deprived, you may also suffer from depression. Yet the steroids and cortisone topical creams often recommended provide only temporary relief, while worsening the problem long-term, since the skin is progressively thinned by them.

Not knowing what leads to a flare-up keeps sufferers on edge. Any provocation, physical or emotional, can throw you off and result in itching and irritation.

The bottom line is that eczema-prone DSPWs need to avoid irritating ingredients *and* irritating life situations. Cultivate calm, meditate, and have a cup of anti-inflammatory green tea. One brand calls their green tea "Zen." No one needs it more than you.


## A COMPLEX SKIN TYPE

DSPW is one of the most challenging and complex of the Baumann Skin Types because you have (or have the potential for) every kind of skin problem.

Your skin is dry, putting you at risk for eczema and related dry skin conditions. Your skin is sensitive, causing redness, irritation, stinging, and rashes in reaction to many skin care ingredients and other provocations. Your skin is pigmented, producing freckles, brown spots, and sun spots. And your skin is wrinkled; so that later in life, you are likely to get wrinkles and show the signs of aging more than certain other types.

The way these factors interact is highly individual, and what manifests for you will depend on how you score in each of the four categories. Dryness combined with skin sensitivity can result in acne, rosacea, and eczema. For more information on how your scores interact to create your particular skin problems, you may wish to reread Chapter Two.

Fortunately, the right regimen can help. But given all of these possible skin issues, there is no single prescription, so I have created a number of different and individualized skin care regimens, which you can find in a later section of this chapter.

Wrinkling may result from genetics, lifestyle factors (like sunning and smoking), diet, or any combination of these factors. In some people, eczema may result from an autoimmune condition. Therefore, some eczema sufferers find that sun exposure helps their skin, because it can downshift the hyperreactivity of the autoimmune response. But sunbathing to control eczema can increase skin's wrinkling and dryness, further contributing to eczema. Sun exposure and hot climates will also worsen rosacea.

Is there anything good about your skin? Well, your risk for non-melanoma skin cancer may be lower than many other types. However, please consult "How to Recognize a Non-Melanoma Skin Cancer" in Chapter Seven to learn to distinguish potentially harmful signs—and make sure to go to a dermatologist for annual checkups in any case.

## A CLOSE-UP LOOK AT YOUR SKIN

With DSPW skin you may experience any of the following:

- Dryness and flaking
- Itching skin
- Pink scaled patches
- Dark patches and spots in response to injury or trauma
- Facial redness and flushing
- Broken blood vessels in the face
- Acne
- Dark circles under the eyes
- Increased susceptibility to skin allergies
- Dry lips
- Skin darkening at irritated areas, such as the back of the knees and inside of the elbows

Both light- and dark-skinned people can be DSPWs. Lighter-skin-toned DSPWs may suffer from dark spots, melasma, or freckles from previous sun exposure. Please refer to the section on pigmentation in Chapter Two to learn more about melasma and see if you might have it.

Melasma can be treated with bleaching creams, but it's most effective to stop taking any form of hormones (like birth control pills or HRT), as they tend to increase pigmentation. Avoid sun exposure since that will worsen it. Choose the right sunscreen because some products fail to block UVA rays, which contribute to melasma. Wear a UVA-blocking sunscreen indoors, and even in a car or on an airplane, because UVA rays penetrate glass. The good news about melasma is that it tends to improve after menopause.

Although darker-toned DSPWs do not freckle, they have complex issues for other reasons. Darker-skinned people often get dark patches after inflammation. Once the redness and itching has gone, it's replaced by a dark patch, which can last, increasing irritation and dryness.

On darker skin, flaking dry skin may look like gray scales. Many people call this "ashy skin" and several skin care products are marketed to address it—though it's simply dryness and can be treated with any good moisturizer. Choose the right body product or face cream, depending on where the dryness occurs.

## ADJUSTING YOUR SKIN CARE

Your ideal climate is humid. In the winter, the drop in humidity may increase dryness and skin sensitivity, leading to skin scaling and itching. Drying environments, such as airplanes or desert locales, can further dehydrate your thirsty skin. DSPWs may also develop dryness, itching, and increased sensitivity to heavy winter clothes made from fabrics like wool, because they rub against and irritate the skin.

You need to alter your skin care regimen with the seasons. Don't just blindly stick to one regimen. Pay attention to your skin's condition, and adjust as needed. In dry climates, moisturize more frequently, using a heavier cream product. In more humid locales, you can get away with a lighter product. When dark spots develop, treat them, and when they leave, return to a maintenance program. Later in this chapter, I'll offer you several options.

For DSPWs, skin problems will often increase with age. After forty, skin dryness can worsen, especially in women going through menopause, requiring frequent moisturizing and richer moisturizers. Skin sensitivity increases with age, because as you are exposed to more topical skin care ingredients, more allergies can develop—until you reach your eighties and nineties, when allergies lessen due to diminished immune function. Therefore, find a few products that work for you and stick with them. Freckles, sun spots, visible blood vessels (sometimes seen with rosacea), and wrinkles also worsen with age, while acne and melasma tend to lessen. With your range of skin problems, I can't promise a permanent solution, but I can promise improvement if you stick with the strategies I'll offer in the next section of this chapter.

**Dr. Baumann's Bottom Line:** Your skin options must be right on the money. You have no room for error, so follow my advice to a T. If you think that you suffer from eczema, see your dermatologist. In many cases of eczema, moisturizers and routine skin care are not enough. Luckily, new prescription medications such as Elidel are very effective at treating this condition.

## EVERYDAY CARE FOR YOUR SKIN

The goal of your skin care routine is to address skin dryness, skin sensitivity, and dark spots with products that deliver ingredients that hydrate your skin, decrease its sensitivity, and reduce dark spots. Your daily regimen will also help to rebuild the skin barrier, lessen inflammation, prevent and treat wrinkles, and prevent and treat acne.

Because DSPW skin can potentially suffer from so many different kinds of problems, adjust your regimen to your skin's current condition. Here you'll find regimens to use if you are experiencing dark spots, redness and stinging, or acne.

If you suffer from acne, it is best to see a dermatologist. Ingredients in over-the-counter acne products such as benzoyl peroxide and salicylic acid will only further dry and irritate your skin. Your dermatologist can prescribe sulfur-containing and antibiotic topical medications or even oral medications that can treat your acne without irritating your skin. Light treatments (*not* sun exposure, which can worsen acne) can be useful as well.

If your skin problems are troublesome, I suggest you try your regimen for only two weeks, or until you can get into a dermatologist's office. Make your appointment today.

**DAILY SKIN CARE**

### REGIMEN FOR TREATING DARK SPOTS:

| AM | PM |
|---|---|
| Step 1: Wash with a cleanser | Step 1: Wash with a cleanser |
| Step 2: Rinse with facial water | Step 2: Rinse with facial water |
| Step 3: Apply a lightening gel | Step 3: Apply a lightening gel |
| Step 4: Apply a moisturizer with sunscreen | Step 4: Apply an antioxidant-containing night cream |

|           AM           |           PM           |
| --- | --- |

Step 5: Apply a foundation with
    sunscreen (optional)

In the morning, wash your face with a cold cream or oil cleanser, which is less drying than other cleansers. Rinse your face with facial water. (See pages 198–199 for more information on facial water.) Then quickly apply a lightening gel to your dark spots, and next apply a moisturizer containing SPF. Try to apply the moisturizer while your face is still moist to trap water in your skin. Finally, use a foundation with SPF, if you wish.

    In the evening, wash with a cold cream or oil cleanser, then rinse with facial water. Apply a lightening gel to dark spots, then quickly apply a night cream containing antioxidants.

    If you have acne, you can also follow this regimen, plus add a sulfur-containing mask once or twice a week. Apply the mask after cleansing, leave it on as per the instructions, and wash it off. Then continue with the rest of the regimen.

## REGIMEN FOR MAINTENANCE ONCE DARK SPOTS HAVE CLEARED:

|           AM           |           PM           |
| --- | --- |

Step 1: Wash with cleanser

Step 2: Apply antioxidant serum

Step 3: Spray facial water

Step 4: Apply an SPF-containing
    moisturizer and/or sunscreen

Step 5: Apply a foundation with
    sunscreen (optional)

Step 1: Wash with cleanser

Step 2: Spray facial water

Step 3: Apply antioxidant-
    containing cream

In the morning, wash your face with cleanser. You can use a cold cream, facial oil, or soothing cleanser or lotion. Next, apply an antioxidant serum. Spray facial water, then quickly apply a moisturizer-containing SPF. Finally, apply a foundation with SPF.

    In the evening, wash with the same cleanser and spray facial water. While your skin is still moist, apply an antioxidant-containing night cream.

## REGIMEN FOR USE AFTER SPOTS HAVE CLEARED BUT WHEN YOU HAVE REDNESS AND STINGING:

| AM | PM |
| --- | --- |
| Step 1: Wash with cleanser | Step 1: Wash with cleanser |
| Step 2: Rinse with facial water | Step 2: Rinse with facial water |
| Step 3: Apply anti-inflammatory product | Step 3: Apply anti-inflammatory product |
| Step 4: Apply an SPF-containing moisturizer and/or sunscreen | Step 4: Apply antioxidant-containing cream |
| Step 5: Apply a foundation with sunscreen (optional) | Step 5: Once or twice a week use a sulfur-containing mask |

In the morning, wash with your choice of cleanser and rinse with facial water. Apply an anti-inflammatory product (see the list on the following page). Next, apply moisturizer with SPF, and follow with a foundation containing SPF if you wish.

In the evening, wash with cleanser and rinse with facial water. Apply the same anti-inflammatory product, then a night cream containing antioxidants.

Once or twice a week, use a mask containing sulfur. Apply the mask after cleansing, leave it or as per the instructions, and wash it off. Then continue with the rest of the regimen.

## Cleansers

DSPWs should avoid any cleansers that foam. Best for you are oil-based cleansers or cold creams.

### RECOMMENDED CLEANSERS

$ Aveeno Positively Radiant Daily Cleansing Pads
$ Eucerin Redness Relief Soothing Cleanser
$ Elemis Chamomile Cleaning Milk

$ Quintessence Skin Science Purifying Cleanser
$$ Clarins Extra-Comfort Cleansing Cream
$$ Elizabeth Arden Millenium Hydrating Cleanser
$$ Paula's Choice Skin Recovery Cleanser
$$ Estée Lauder Soft Clean Tender Creme Cleanser
$$ La Roche-Posay Toleriane Dermo-Cleanser
$$ Murad Essential-C Cleanser
$$ Nia24 Gentle Cleansing Cream
$$ VMV Hypoallergenics Moisture Rich Creammmy Cleansing Milk
$$$ Darphin Intral Cleansing Milk

**Baumann's Choice:** VMV Hypoallergenics Moisture Rich Creammmy Cleansing Milk because it does not contain allergens that could irritate your sensitive skin

### RECOMMENDED COLD CREAMS AND OIL CLEANSERS FOR VERY DRY SKIN

$ Avene Cold Cream for very dry sensitive skin
$ Pond's Cold Cream
$$ DHC Cleansing Oil
$$ Shu Uemura Cleansing Beauty Oil Premium A/O
$$ SK II Facial Treatment Cleansing Oil
$$ Laura Mercier Purifying Oil—Light or Rich
$$$ Clinique Take The Day Off Cleansing Balm

**Baumann's Choice:** Shu Uemura Cleansing Beauty Oil Premium A/O because it contains green tea

## Anti-Inflammatory Products

Anti-inflammatory products are often serums and gels. While the most effective ones are prescription products, a few over-the-counter options are available.

### RECOMMENDED ANTI-INFLAMMATORY PRODUCTS

$ Eucerin Redness Relief Daily Perfecting Lotion
$ Paula's Choice Skin Relief Treatment
$$$ Combray by Solenne
$$$ B. Kamins Booster Blue Rosacea Treatment
$$$ Pevonia Rose RS2 Concentrate

**Baumann's Choice:** Paula's Choice Skin Relief Treatment has willow herb.

## Antioxidant Serums

Use these antioxidant serums as called for in some of the regimens unless you experience frequent redness and stinging in response to skin care products. If so, they're too irritating for you.

### RECOMMENDED ANTIOXIDANT SERUMS

- $  Neutrogena Ageless Restoratives Anti-Oxidant Booster Serum
- $$  Olay Professional ProX Skin Tightening Serum
- $$  Josie Maran 100% Organic Argan Oil
- $$  Caudalie Vinoperfect Complexion Correcting Radiance Serum
- $$  Wai Hope Private Reserve Serum di Hope
- $$$  Combray Serum

**Baumann's Choice:** Wai Hope Private Reserve Serum di Hope because it contains many organic antioxidants

## Facial Water

A DSPW should never use toners, which usually have drying ingredients designed to remove lipids from the skin. Your skin needs all the lipids it can get. Toners also contain ingredients that will further irritate your sensitive skin.

If your skin is supersensitive, it may benefit from special waters. In a recent study, skin that was irritated by detergent cleared faster when rinsed with $CO_2$-enriched tap water for one minute once daily, as compared to rinsing with regular tap water. This result suggests that washing your face with Pellegrino or another carbonated water may be beneficial. You may find this impractical, but it is an interesting idea.

Spray facial water on your face just before applying eye cream and moisturizer. The moisturizer and eye cream will help trap the water on the skin, giving the skin a reservoir to pull water from. This is particularly beneficial in low-humidity environments such as the dry winter air or an airplane.

Facial waters come from thermal springs. They do not contain chemicals such as chlorine that are added to our tap water to keep it free from algae and other organisms. The constituents of the water vary according to the source. Vichy water contains sulfur, while the La Roche-Posay water contains selenium and has been shown to be effective in treating eczema. Both selenium and sulfur can be anti-inflammatory.

## RECOMMENDED FACIAL WATERS

- $ Twinlab Na-Pca Non Oily with Aloe Vera
- $$ Avène Thermal Water Spray
- $$ Wai Hope Seawater Recharging Mist
- $$ Fresh Rose Marigold Tonic Water
- $$ La Roche-Posay Thermal Spring Water
- $$ Depsea Water Mist, chamomile
- $$ Vichy Thermal Spa Water
- $$$ Susan Ciminelli Seawater

**Baumann's Choice:** La Roche-Posay Thermal Spring Water contains selenium, which soothes the skin.

## Treatments for Dark Spots

I really prefer prescription products for lightening dark spots, but here are some suggestions if you want to try over-the-counter products.

## RECOMMENDED LIGHTENING PRODUCTS

- $ Topix HQS-2 Skin Lightening Cream
- $ Porcelana Fade Dark Spots Nighttime Treatment
- $ Skineffects by Dr. Jeffrey Dover Advanced Brightening Complex
- $$ Elure Advanced Whitening Lotion For Face and Neck
- $$ PCA Skin pHaze 23 A&C Synergy Serum
- $$ Clinique Clinical Even Better Dark Spot Corrector
- $$$ Dr. Brandt Flaws No More Lightening Serum
- $$$ SkinCeuticals Phyto + Botanical Gel for Hyperpigmentation
- $$$ Vivite Vibrance Therapy

**Baumann's Choice:** The soon-to-be-released Elure Advanced Whitening Lotion For Face and Neck contains a new ingredient to break down skin melanin and even skin tone.

## Moisturizers

Apply moisturizer frequently throughout the day—in the morning after gently cleansing your face, again in the later afternoon or early evening, and finally at bedtime. With a very low O/D score, or during times of low humidity, use creams rather than lotions. Your skin needs the extra moisture. If you have a medium O/D score of 17–26, or during times of high humidity when you prefer a lighter product, use lotions. Avoid heavily fragranced moisturizers and those containing essential oils.

### RECOMMENDED DAYTIME MOISTURIZERS (WITH SPF)

$ Aveeno Positively Radiant Daily Moisturizer (with soy)
$ Aveeno Ultra-Calming Daily Moisturizer SPF 15
$ Avon Anew Ultimate Age Repair Day Cream SPF 25
$ Neutrogena Healthy Skin Visibly Even Daily SPF 15 Moisturizer
$ Olay Complete Defense Daily UV Moisturizer SPF 30
$$ Canyon Ranch Your Transformation Protect UVA/UVB Facial Moisturizer
$$ Elizabeth Arden Intervene Radiance Boosting Moisture Cream SPF 15
$$ Clinique Even Better Skin Tone Correcting Moisturizer SPF 20
$$ Patricia Wexler M.D. Dermatology Brightening Moisturizer
$$ Vichy Capital Soleil Hydra-Cream Face 50+

**Baumann's Choice:** Clinique Even Better Skin Tone Correcting Moisturizer SPF 20

### RECOMMENDED NIGHTTIME MOISTURIZERS

$ Ageless Vitality Elasticity Recharging System Restorative Night Treatment
$ Burt's Bees Healthy Treatment Marshmallow Vanishing Creme
$ Eucerin Redness Relief Soothing Night Creme
$ Bamboo Leaf Ultra Soothing Anti-Redness Cream
$$ Atopalm MLE Face Cream
$$ Kiehl's Creme d'Elegance Repairateur
$$ La Roche-Posay Toleriane Soothing Protective Facial Cream
$$ Nia24 Intensive Recovery Complex

$$$  Bobbi Brown Intensive Skin Supplement
$$$  Erno Laszlo Total Skin Revitalizer

**Baumann's Choice:** Atopalm MLE Face Cream is very hydrating and contains pseudoceramide to help repair the skin barrier.

## Eye Creams

You have enough skin problems already, so why not make life easy and skip the eye cream? Instead you can apply your regular moisturizer around the eyes. If you really want to try one, select one of these products and apply it prior to moisturizer.

### RECOMMENDED EYE CREAMS

$  Neutrogena Visibly Firm Eye Cream
$$  Obagi Nu-Derm Eye Cream
$$  Nia24 Eye Repair Complex
$$  Clinique All About Eyes Rich
$$$  Bobbi Brown Extra Repair Cream

**Baumann's Choice:** Neutrogena Visibly Firm Eye Cream. (When I travel, to save space, I use this as my facial night cream as well.)

## Masks

Here are recommended masks containing sulfur, as called for in two of the nonprescription regimens.

### RECOMMENDED SULFUR-CONTAINING MASKS

$$  DDF Sulfur Therapeutic Mask
$$  Peter Thomas Roth Sulfur Cooling Masque

## Exfoliation

DSPWs should never exfoliate since it can make your skin more sensitive and hurt your skin barrier. Concentrate instead on moisturizing.

## SHOPPING FOR PRODUCTS

Reading product labels is particularly important for DSPWs, whose sensitive skin can be irritated by so many types of ingredients. Other ingredients are beneficial, so you should choose products containing them. Below, I've listed ingredients that are helpful for preventing and treating dark spots, hydrating the skin, improving wrinkles, and preventing inflammation—as well as ingredients to avoid. If you find skin care products that are not on my lists, please share them with me at www.skintypesolutions.com.

---

### SKIN CARE INGREDIENTS TO USE

#### To improve dark spots:

- Arbutin
- Cucumber extract
- *Glycyrrhiza glabra* (licorice extract)
- Hydroquinone
- Kojic acid
- Magnesium ascorbyl phosphate
- Mulberry extract
- Tyrostat

#### To prevent dark spots:

- *Cocos nucifera* (coconut extract), unless you have acne
- Cucumber
- Niacinamide
- Pycnogenol (a pine bark extract)
- *Saxifraga sarmentosa* extract (strawberry begonia)

#### To moisturize and hydrate:

- *Ajuga turkestanica*
- Aloe vera
- Apricot kernel oil
- Borage seed oil
- Canola oil
- Ceramide
- Cholesterol
- Cocoa butter (not if you have acne)
- Colloidal oatmeal
- Dexpanthenol (provitamin $B_5$)
- Dimethicone
- Evening primrose oil
- Glycerin
- Jojoba oil
- Macadamia nut oil
- Olive oil
- Safflower oil
- Shea butter

### To prevent wrinkles:

- Basil
- Caffeine
- *Camilla sinensis* (green tea, white tea)
- Carrot extract
- Coenzyme Q$_{10}$ (ubiquinone)
- Copper peptide
- Curcumin (tetrahydracurcumin or turmeric)
- Ferulic acid
- Feverfew
- Ginger
- Ginseng
- Grape seed extract
- Idebenone
- Lutein
- Lycopene
- *Punica granatum* (pomegranate)
- Pycnogenol (a pine bark extract)
- Rosemary
- Silymarin
- Yucca

### To improve wrinkles:

- Copper peptide
- *Ginkgo biloba*
- Vitamin C (ascorbic acid), may be too irritating for you

### Anti-inflammatory:

- Aloe vera
- Chamomile
- Colloidal oatmeal
- Cucumber
- Dexpanthenol (provitamin B$_5$)
- *Epibolium angustifolium* (willow herb)
- Evening primrose oil
- Feverfew
- Green tea
- Licochalone
- Mirabilis
- Perilla leaf extract
- Pycnogenol (a pine bark extract)
- Red algae
- Thyme
- *Trifolium pretense* (red clover)
- Zinc

## SKIN CARE PRODUCTS TO AVOID

### For all DSPWs:

- Cleansing products that foam
- Scrubs
- Toners

### If you have acne:

- Butyl stearate
- Cinnamon oil
- Cocoa butter
- *Cocos nucifera* (coconut oil)
- Decyl oleate
- Isopropyl isostearate
- Isopropyl myristate
- Isopropyl palmitate
- Isostearyl neopentanoate
- Lanolin
- Myristyl myristate
- Myristyl propionate
- Octyl palmitate or isocetyl stearate
- Octyl stearate
- Peppermint oil
- Propylene glycol-2 (PPG-2)

### If you have skin redness:

- Alpha hydroxy acids (lactic acid, glycolic acid)
- Alpha lipoic acid
- Benzoyl peroxide
- Gluconolactone
- Phytic acid
- Polyhydroxy acids
- Retinaldehyde
- Retinol
- Retinyl palmitate
- Vitamin C (ascorbic acid)

# SUN PROTECTION FOR YOUR SKIN

Use creams. If you have dark spots, there are a few sunscreens with depigmenting agents, such as Philosophy A Pigment of Your Imagination. When possible, look for sunscreens that also contain antioxidants.

## RECOMMENDED SUN PROTECTION PRODUCTS

$ Blue Lizard Sunscreen Sensitive SPF 30
$ Eucerin Q10 Anti-Wrinkle Sensitive Skin Lotion SPF 15

$   Aveeno Ultra-Calming Moisturizing Lotion with SPF 30

$$   Topix Glycolix Elite Sunscreen SPF 30

$$   SkinCeuticals Ultimate UV Defense SPF 30

$$$   Darphin Vital Protection Age-Defying Protective Lotion SPF 50

$$   Kiehl's Abyssine Cream + SPF 23

$$$   Perricone MD More Than Moisture SPF 30

$$$   Natura Bisse NB Ceutical Daily Defense Oil-Free Fluid SPF 30

$$$   Sisley Broad Spectrum Sunscreen, SPF 40

**Baumann's Choice:** Blue Lizard Sunscreen Sensitive SPF 30 because it is chemical free

## PROCEDURES FOR YOUR SKIN TYPE

There are no procedures that can improve the dryness and sensitivity of your skin. These problems are best treated with skin care products, life-style changes, and dietary recommendations. Please go to www.skintype solutions.com for my nutritional recommendations. However, your dark spots can be treated and there are more options to get rid of wrinkles than ever before.

## Lasers and Light Treatments

For DSPWs with light skin, a number of types of lasers and light treatments are specifically designed to remove brown spots such as freckles.

Lasers and light treatments work by targeting a particular color. For ex-ample, pigmented lesion lasers such as the Ruby laser, the Alexandrite laser, or the Nd:Yag emit a specific wavelength of light that can only be absorbed by the color brown. The Intense Pulsed Light treatments emit different wavelengths of light that target several skin features, such as dark spots and blood vessels.

When the laser or light is focused on a brown spot, the brown pigment (melanin) absorbs the energy of the light until the pigment becomes so hot that the cells containing melanin burst. The surrounding non-melanin-containing cells are unharmed. Patients with darker skin cannot use this technology because their normal skin cells contain higher amounts of melanin and would also be affected.

## Chemical Peels

DSPWs with darker skin can use light chemical peels on their dark spots. Glycolic acid– and lactic acid–containing peels are best for your type because they hydrate the skin as well as exfoliating it. In addition, these peels have been shown to improve fine wrinkles. Although you can get these alpha hydroxy acid peels at a salon, a dermatologist will be able to use a higher concentration of AHA, giving you better results.

## Dermal Fillers

There are many good dermal fillers available to treat wrinkles. I prefer those containing collagen or hyaluronic acid. These fillers are ideal for DSPWs (and DSNWs) because collagen and hyaluronic acid are naturally occurring substances that look and feel natural and give instantaneous results.

## ONGOING CARE FOR YOUR SKIN

Your skin may seem high maintenance now, but with a clear plan and these easy-to-follow regimens, you can finally manage your skin. Avoid cleansers that foam. Instead use an oil-based cleanser or a cold cream. Moisturize at least twice a day. Apply sunscreen daily, and use more often (reapplying hourly) if you are out in the sun.

# CHAPTER THIRTEEN

# Dry, Sensitive, Pigmented, and Tight: DSPT

## BAUMANN SKIN TYPE NUMBER 1

∎

*"I know I need to moisturize, but there are so many choices. Are there any that will prevent my skin sensitivity and the resulting dark patches? If I need more than one product, do I use the light-ening product first or the moisturizer?"*

## ABOUT YOUR SKIN

If your questionnaire results reveal you as a DSPT, you probably face a variety of skin issues. Your skin can be prone to eczema, dryness, acne, flaking, redness, itching, and rosacea. The problems that plague DSPTs are more than visually disturbing. Having itchy skin, redness, rosacea, or acne is just plain uncomfortable. You can't forget about it. It's a constant irritation and distraction. DSPTs feel helpless in managing their skin's dryness and sensitivity. Remember the old expression "Walk a mile in my shoes"? Well, most other Skin Types wouldn't want to spend a day in your skin. And few people can imagine the ongoing distress that DSPTs experience every minute of their lives.

Even though your reddened, dry, and flaky skin cries out for moisturizers, your skin's sensitivity produces reactions to so many ingredients that you don't feel confident trying out products. Fragrance in skin care products, detergents in soaps, rough fabrics, and blustery weather can cause disturbances. Heavy moisturizers may cause acne. What can you feel happy about? Well, your risk for non-melanoma skin cancer may be slightly lower than for other types, but it is always best to get regular checkups.

All four Dry, Sensitive Skin Types have a disturbed skin barrier. To learn how dryness, sensitivity, and pigmentation interact to create the skin issues you experience, please read "A Disturbed Skin Barrier" in Chapter Twelve. Many people of medium-tone skin have the DSPT type, which includes people of Latin American, Spanish, Mediterranean, or Middle Eastern ancestry. This type is also quite common among African Americans and Asians.

## DEALING WITH DRYNESS

Many DSPTs are people of color for whom skin dryness can lead to flaking and "ashiness," an appearance of grayness that occurs because as dry skin flakes off, it whitens, while the dark skin tone shows through underneath. As companies market products to prevent "ashiness," remember it's another name for dryness, which can be addressed with the right moisturizers.

Dark-skin-toned DSPTs may have dry, sensitive skin for genetic reasons, but their skin's dryness can also result from environmental conditions and chemical exposures. Many of the products and chemical treatments used on black hair can undermine the skin barrier and contribute to allergies.

An allergy occurs when the immune system makes antibodies that react to a substance. For example, some people have antibodies to poison ivy and they develop a rash when exposed to it, while others do not have this antibody and don't react to it. Ingredients can penetrate a compromised skin barrier to reach the bloodstream, where they can produce an allergic reaction. Irritant rashes are different, though often confused with allergies. An irritating substance causes a skin rash but, unlike an allergy, is not caused by antibodies. An impaired skin barrier makes you more susceptible.

Rashes, redness, and itching are all responses to inflammation, which further undermines the skin barrier. Once your skin is inflamed, you need to calm it by avoiding irritants and accessing skin soothers. Continued damage can lead to eczema, to which DSPTs are prone.

## DSPTs AND ECZEMA

Over twelve million people have eczema, also known as atopic dermatitis (AD), a severe form of dry skin that tends to recur in the same place, such as behind the knees, on the wrists, knuckles, and ankles, and in the bend of the arm. It begins as an itching patch that becomes red and inflamed. Scratching the area can cause the skin to tear and become infected. In

DSPT and DSPW Types, the affected areas become dark and can take months to fade to your natural skin color. Eczema results from a combination of dryness and sensitivity, and sometimes allergies play a part. These may include both topical allergies to substances that touch the skin and internal reactions to foods, inhalants, and other substances that produce an allergic reaction via the skin.

## Do I Have Eczema?

If you have any of the following symptoms, you may have eczema:

- Itching skin anywhere on the face or body
- Irritation and the need to frequently scratch behind the knees, elbows, wrists, or ankles
- Areas of itching turn into darkened or reddened patches that remain after itching has calmed
- Cracking of the skin over areas of redness and dryness, especially over joints
- Itching and redness that tend to recur in the same areas of the body
- Itching, redness, and scaling behind the ears
- History of allergies or asthma in you or your family

One key rule is that it's important not to scratch when you feel the itch because the friction of scratching further degrades the skin barrier. Instead I'll provide you with both over-the-counter and prescription medications to calm eczema flares.

## Predisposed to Eczema?

Eczema can often be an inherited condition, striking people with a family history or medical history of asthma and allergies. The onset of eczema usually occurs within the first year of life and most people who are going to get it develop it by age five. Luckily, many "grow out of it," plagued in the future by just routine dry skin. Adults with atopic dermatitis usually have excessively sensitive skin.

A recent study reveals that breast-fed infants have a lower incidence of atopic dermatitis, most likely because breast-fed infants are not exposed to common allergens like dairy products and soy before their young immune systems have developed. Interestingly, another study showed that babies who were breast-fed by mothers who eliminated common allergenic foods (such as eggs, dairy, fish, peanuts, and soybeans) from their diets had a lower incidence of eczema than breast-fed babies whose mothers were not on restricted diets.

## Avoiding Irritants

The three key interventions for addressing both dryness and eczema are:

- Calming inflammation
- Rebuilding the barrier
- Hydrating the skin

Although there is no cure for eczema, it can be controlled. It's important to avoid sun exposure and use skin care products designed to strengthen the skin's barrier. My selections will include ingredients that hydrate the skin and repair the skin's barrier, allowing the skin to better hold on to water.

## DSPT ENVIRONMENTAL IMPACT REPORT

The problems DSPTs suffer also change with the seasons, as weather conditions can assault your dry, sensitive skin. It's hard to say which season is best for your Dry, Pigmented Skin Type. In the summer, sun exposure may darken dark spots. As a result, sun protection and skin lightening are often needed. When the temperature drops, so do humidity levels, with wintry cold and low humidity increasing dryness and skin sensitivity. Heavy winter clothes, made with rough fabrics like wool, may cause skin friction that worsens dryness and sensitivity. For DSPTs, the ideal climate is a cool, humid environment. Moving to Arizona is not recommended.

## A CLOSE-UP LOOK AT YOUR SKIN

With DSPT skin you may experience any of the following:

- Eczema (atopic dermatitis)
- Scaling skin
- Thick rough patches of skin
- Itching

- Dryness that worsens in winter or low-humidity climates
- Sensitivity to fragrances that can cause skin rashes
- Dryness from detergents, creating "dishpan hands"
- Dark patches in areas of inflammation or trauma such as after a cut
- Dark patches in area of sun exposure
- Dark eyelids
- Dark circles under the eyes

With tight skin, you won't experience that much wrinkling as you age, while other problems *will* worsen with aging. Your dry skin gets drier as the years go by. Winter is harder on skin than in youth, resulting in redness, flaking, and cracking. Going without a moisturizer is usually not an option over the age of fifty. Heavier night creams will feel good to older DSPTs; however, don't be fooled into buying expensive ones with antiaging ingredients you don't need. I'll offer the right moisturizers later in this chapter. For women, melasma and dark spots will improve with declining estrogen levels in perimenopause and menopause. However, lower estrogen levels also contribute to dry skin. In the eighties and nineties, as the immune system weakens, any condition arising from allergies or autoimmune conditions (such as certain cases of eczema) may improve.

## ETHNICITY AND DSPT SKIN

Many DSPT Asians have a higher incidence of eczema and melasma, but a lower incidence of wrinkles and skin cancer than do Caucasians. As a result, Asian product lines focus more closely on treating dryness and pigmentation. Due to biochemical differences, Asian skin also reacts differently to products than Caucasian and black skin.

For example, several studies have demonstrated that Japanese skin is more reactive to detergents. This may be why many Asians prefer oil-based cleansers. While detergents (contained in most cleansers, shampoos, face and body soaps, laundry and dish-cleaning products) are drying and should be avoided by all Dry, Sensitive Types, those of Asian ancestry in particular should steer clear of soaps, shampoos, and cleaning products that vigorously foam. Pick milder products, rinse thoroughly after cleansing, and re-moisturize after use. Also wear rubber gloves when using household cleaning products. Although I recommend skin care products that contain hydroquinone, an ingredient used in skin care to lighten dark spots, some Asians with dry, sensitive skin and a history of ochronosis (a hereditary enzyme deficiency) should avoid it, as they may develop the blackish patches characteristic of this condition.

Instead, Asian DSPTs can receive hydroquinone-free peels, light treatments, or microdermabrasion from a dermatologist or spa professional. I recommend you request a "light" rather than strong treatment, proceeding gradually to assure that your skin does not become irritated.

## PRODUCT CHOICES FOR DSPT SKIN

DSPTs benefit from constant moisturizer use, and you also need products and treatments that lighten dark patches and melasma. However, DSPTs react negatively to a wide range of products and ingredients. Fragrances are the most common allergens, instigating rashes more than anything else, including parabens and other chemical preservatives used in skin care. Obviously, you should avoid dousing yourself in perfume, although you may be able to find a single essential oil that does not cause a reaction. Still, the search to find one can create so much havoc, it may not be worth it. As mentioned earlier, most skin care products, even those marketed as fragrance free, contain some perfume to mask the unpleasant smell of the ingredients. The perfume used for this purpose is often a mix containing as many as forty or more different ingredients, so identifying the culprit can be next to impossible. One patient of mine developed a rash from the perfume samples stapled inside magazines. Now before she reads a magazine, she asks her boyfriend to remove the offending samples.

Not knowing which ingredients cause reactions makes skin care shopping a danger-fraught experience. You may find that when you use your new skin purchases, your skin flares up with rashes and redness that can persist for days, weeks, and months. Don't think that you can use the cream you bought on a less critical area, like your hands, feet, or legs. When you're at risk for eczema, you have to be ultracareful. Many DSPT patients report that it's an achievement to find even a single product that they can safely use.

## THE MOISTURE CURE

DSPTs, if I have one message to you, it's this: Hydrate, hydrate, hydrate.

Moisturizers with an SPF factor blended into simple beneficial ingredients, like shea butter, cocoa butter, olive and jojoba oils, are best for you.

Your skin care products should either contain or cause the skin to produce ceramides, fatty acids, and cholesterol. These three different forms of fat are needed to create a healthy skin barrier. In addition, you must apply a moisturizer at least twice a day. Notice that I said *at least*. In your case, more is better. I also advise you to use both a sunscreen and a moisturizer, because sunscreens alone will not provide enough hydration. Heavy night creams are good but should not contain fragrances that will further irritate and dry your skin. Beware of the expensive creams that do contain fragrances. Sunscreens must be worn daily, for two reasons. First, the sun disrupts the skin's barrier; and second, the sun causes dark spots.

Unfortunately, there are no in-office dermatological procedures that I know of that will improve the skin's barrier. In many cases, dark spots in lighter-skinned individuals can be treated with laser and light therapies. Both dark- and light-skinned individuals may be treated with chemical peels or microdermabrasion to hasten the resolution of dark spots and to temporarily improve the roughness of the skin. Prescription medications can be used to treat eczema flare-ups and to lighten dark spots. But above all, you must take control and be vigilant about moisturizing your skin and avoiding irritants.

**Dr. Baumann's Bottom Line:** For you, moisturizing as often as four times a day isn't too much. Apply moisturizers immediately after bathing, dishwashing, or facing the elements. Do it whenever you change clothes. You cannot over-moisturize your skin.

## EVERYDAY CARE FOR YOUR SKIN

The goal of your skin care routine is to heal your skin's barrier to make it stronger, helping it hold on to moisture (so that your skin becomes less dry) and keep out allergens and irritants (so that your skin becomes less sensitive). To accomplish these goals, you'll use products that deliver barrier repair ingredients. This will also help prevent inflammation that leads to dark spots. In addition, your daily regimen will also help to prevent and treat acne.

While not everyone with this type will get acne, having dry skin does not protect you from outbreaks. I'll provide optional treatments for pimples.

Products designed for "sensitive skin" are for dry, sensitive types. However, if you have a high P/N score (over 30), there are few sensitive skin products that contain depigmenting agents. I will point you toward products that will give your skin an even tone in addition to hydrating it, building its barrier, and decreasing its sensitivity.

## DAILY SKIN CARE

### REGIMEN

| AM | PM |
|---|---|
| Step 1: Wash with cleanser | Step 1: Wash with cleanser |
| Step 2: Spray facial water | Step 2: Spray facial water |
| Step 3: Apply eye cream (optional) | Step 3: Apply eye cream (optional) |
| Step 4: Apply skin lightener to spots (optional) | Step 4: Apply skin lightener to spots (optional) |
| Step 5: Apply moisturizer | Step 5: Apply moisturizer |
| Step 6: Apply sunscreen | |
| Step 7: Apply foundation (optional) | |

In the morning, wash your face with a cleanser, then spray on facial water. Eye cream use is optional, you can use one if you want. In that case, be prepared to apply your eye cream, skin lightener, and moisturizer in rapid sequence while your face is still damp from the facial water. Have all your products out and ready for use to assure you apply them all before your face dries. If the water evaporates prior to moisturizer application, this will dry your skin, which is totally counterproductive. Skin lightener should be applied to dark spots only. Then apply moisturizer, sunscreen, and finally, foundation if you wish.

In the evening, wash with a cleanser, spray facial water, and apply an eye cream and a skin lightener if needed. Last, apply moisturizer.

Although you may never before have heard of spraying your face with specially packaged facial waters prior to moisturizing, it's a great secret for hydrating dry skin. You'll find more information about it in this chapter in my section on facial water.

After eight weeks on this regimen, if your dryness and skin sensitivity fail to resolve, try *different* products from my list of recommendations. If your skin still does not improve in another four weeks, see a dermatologist, who can prescribe medication for severe dryness, itching, and eczema that can be used along with this regimen.

# Cleansers

Cleansing and moisturizing are the two most important aspects of your skin regimen. Using the wrong cleanser can aggravate your condition even if you are doing everything else right. Cleansers that contain detergents (which produce a lot of foam and suds) strip your skin of necessary lipids, causing dryness and increased sensitivity. DSPTs should never use soap, shampoo, moisturizer, or hair conditioner that you haven't selected yourself to assure they do not contain irritating ingredients.

Did you know that you can wash your face with oil? It's very popular in Asia, since so many people there have dry skin. If you have acne, this may not work for you; but if you're like me (very dry and scaling), it's a great way to moisturize. I *love* cleansing oils for DSPTs. Try Shu Uemura Cleansing Beauty Oil Premium A/O, being sure to follow the directions that tell you to apply it to a dry face and then add water with your fingertips.

### RECOMMENDED CLEANSERS

- $ Aveeno Positively Radiant Daily Cleansing Pads
- $ Pond's Deep Cleanser Cold Cream (for extremely dry skin)
- $ CeraVe Hydrating Cleanser
- $$ La Roche-Posay Toleriane Dermo-Cleanser
- $$ Babor Cleansing HY-OL
- $$ Moisture Rich Creammmy Cleansing Milk by VMV Hypoallergenics
- $$ Wai Hope Pre Hope Organic Cleanser
- $$$ Darphin Intral Cleansing Milk

**Baumann's Choice:** La Roche-Posay Toleriane Dermo-Cleanser

### RECOMMENDED CLEANSING OILS

- $ Jojoba Cleansing Oil
- $$ M·A·C Cleanse Off Oil
- $$ Shu Uemura Cleansing Beauty Oil Premium A/O
- $$$ Bobbi Brown Cleansing Oil
- $$$ SK-II Cleansing Oil Treatment

**Baumann's Choice:** Shu Uemura Cleansing Beauty Oil Premium A/O

## Facial Water

DSPTs should *never* use toners, which usually have drying ingredients that remove lipids from the skin. Your skin needs all the lipids it can get. Instead of a toner, use a facial water. Spray it on your face immediately prior to applying an eye cream and moisturizer. The moisturizer and eye cream will help trap the water on the skin, giving the skin a reservoir to pull water from. This is especially important in low-humidity environments such as in the winter air, on airplanes, in air-conditioning, or in windy locales.

Facial waters come from thermal springs. They do not contain chemicals such as chlorine that are added to our tap water to keep it free from algae and other organisms. The constituents of the water vary according to the source. Vichy water contains sulfur, while the La Roche-Posay water contains selenium, which has been shown to be effective in treating eczema. Both selenium and sulfur can be anti-inflammatory.

### RECOMMENDED FACIAL WATERS

- $ Evian Mineral Water Spray
- $ La Roche-Posay Thermal Spring Water
- $ Vichy Thermal Spa Water
- $$ Avène Thermal Water Spray
- $$ Chantecaille Pure Rosewater
- $$ Shu Uemura Depsea Water Mist
- $$$ Jurlique Rosewater Spray

**Baumann's Choice:** La Roche-Posay Thermal Spring Water

## Acne Treatment

DSPTs who have acne are a minority, but I haven't forgotten about you. Learning to properly hydrate your skin will actually improve your acne. It is a myth that the skin must be dried out to improve acne. Based on recent studies, dermatologists now believe that acne clears better with a hydrating cleanser than with a drying one. If your acne does not improve, you may add an over-the-counter retinol cream, such as Neutrogena Healthy Skin, followed by a moisturizer in your nighttime regimen. In most cases, this will be enough to clear your skin. If not, please see your dermatologist.

## Treatments for Dark Spots

Any allergenic product can cause inflammation, which in turn can lead to dark spots. When dark spots are present, use a skin lightening gel. Several over-the-counter products are suggested below, but I highly recommend getting a stronger prescription product from your dermatologist.

### RECOMMENDED SKIN LIGHTENERS

- $ Topix HQS-2 Skin Lightening Cream
- $ Porcelana Fade Dark Spots Nighttime Treatment
- $ Skineffects by Dr. Jeffrey Dover Advanced Brightening Complex
- $$ B. Kamins Skin Lightening Treatment
- $$ Elure Advanced Whitening Lotion
- $$ Philosophy A Pigment of Your Imagination
- $$$ Vivite Vibrance Therapy
- $$$ DDF Intensive Holistic Lightener
- $$$ SkinCeuticals Phyto + Botanical Gel for Hyperpigmentation
- $$$ Dr. Brandt Flaws No More Lightening Serum

**Baumann's Choice:** Vivite Vibrance Therapy is one product that is truly worth the cost. Not for those with redness and flushing.

## Moisturizers

You need to moisturize frequently, at least three times daily. The ideal would be in the morning after gently cleansing your face, again in the later afternoon or early evening, and at bedtime. If you have a very low O/D score of 11 to 16, use creams. If you have a medium O/D score of 17 to 26, use lotions. Avoid gels, which are better for oily types.

Assure that every day you are covered with a minimum SPF of 15. You can obtain this degree of protection via a single product, such as moisturizer, or via several used in combination, such as moisturizer and foundation.

### RECOMMENDED EYE CREAMS

- $$ Aveeno Ageless Vitality Elasticity Recharging System-Eye
- $$ DDF Nutrient K Plus
- $$ MD Skincare Lift & Lighten Eye Cream

$$ Philosophy Dark Shadows
$$ Kinerase Pro+Therapy Ultra-Rich Eye Repair
$$$ Sisley Eye and Lip Contour Cream

**Baumann's Choice:** Aveeno Ageless Vitality Elasticity Recharging System-Eye because it contains ingredients that stimulate the skin cells to make elastin. This may help tighten under-eye skin.

## RECOMMENDED DAYTIME MOISTURIZERS

$ Aveeno Positively Radiant Daily Moisturizer SPF 15
$ Good Skin All Calm
$$ Olay Regenerist DNA Superstructure UV Cream - SPF 25
$$ Elizabeth Arden Intervene Moisture Cream SPF 15
$$ Nia24 Sun Damage Prevention 100% Mineral Sunscreen

**Baumann's Choice:** Nia24 Sun Damage Prevention 100% Mineral Sunscreen because it contains niacinamide, green tea, ceramides, and evening primrose

## RECOMMENDED EVENING MOISTURIZERS

$ CeraVe Facial Moisturizing Lotion PM
$ Vaseline Men Body and Face Lotion
$$ Atopalm MLE Cream
$$ Vivite Replenish Hydrating Cream
$$ Nia24 Skin Strengthening Complex Repair Cream
$$ Biotherm Aquasource Biosensitive
$$ Organic Argan Oil
$$ Korres Thyme and Honey Moisturizing Cream
$$ Canyon Ranch Your Transformation Restore Intensive Moisture
$$ Vichy Neovadiol Gf
$$$ Fresh Creme Ancienne
$$$ Kinerase Ultra-Rich Night Repair
$$$ Sisley Botanical Moisturizer with Cucumber
$$$ SK-II Skin Signature Melting Rich Cream

**Baumann's Choice:** CeraVe Facial Moisturizing Lotion PM because it contains ceramides and niacinamide to help reduce inflammation and repair the skin barrier

## Exfoliation

As a rule, people with DSPT skin shouldn't exfoliate, unless your dermatologist recommends it. I have seen many DSPT patients who over-exfoliated, leading to skin redness, tiny red bumps, and inflammation-induced pigmentation. Concentrate instead on moisturizing. Many at-home microdermabrasion kits are available, but I feel you are much better off doing these treatments under the supervision of a dermatologist.

## SHOPPING FOR PRODUCTS

With your sensitive skin, you need to read labels carefully in order to avoid ingredients that may aggravate dryness and pigmentation. Look for ingredients that prevent and improve dark spots, hydrate the skin, and prevent inflammation. If you find favorite products that are not on my recommended lists, please go to www.skintypesolutions.com and share your discoveries with me and others of your Skin Type.

---

**RECOMMENDED SKIN CARE INGREDIENTS**

*To prevent dark spots:*

- *Cocos nucifera* (coconut extract), unless you have acne
- Niacinamide
- Pycnogenol (a pine bark extract)
- Soy, with estrogenic components taken out

*To improve dark spots:*

- Arbutin
- Bearberry extract
- Cucumber extract
- *Glycyrrhiza glabra* (licorice extract)
- Hydroquinone
- Mulberry extract

## To prevent inflammation:

- Aloe vera
- Chamomile
- Colloidal oatmeal
- Cucumber
- Dexpanthenol (provitamin B$_5$)
- *Epilobium angustifolium* (willow herb)
- Evening primrose oil
- Feverfew
- Licochalone
- Perilla leaf extract
- Pycnogenol (a pine bark extract)
- Red algae
- Thyme
- *Trifolium pretense* (red clover)

## To help skin hold on to water:

- Borage seed oil
- Castor oil
- Ceramide
- Cholesterol
- Cocoa butter (avoid if you have acne)
- Colloidal oatmeal
- Dexpanthenol (provitamin B$_5$)
- Dimethicone
- Evening primrose oil
- Glycerin
- Jojoba oil
- Olive oil
- Pumpkin seed oil
- Safflower oil
- Shea butter
- Sunflower oil

### SKIN CARE INGREDIENTS TO AVOID

## Due to irritating detergents:

- Dimethyl dodecyl amido betaine
- Lauryl sulphates
- Sodium dodecyl sulfate
- Sodium laurel sulfate

## Due to increasing acne or skin redness:

- Cinnamon oil
- Cocoa butter
- *Cocos nucifera* (coconut oil)
- Isopropyl isostearate
- Isopropyl myristate
- Peppermint oil

### Due to problematic preservatives:

- Benzalkonium chloride
- Bronopol
- Chlorhexidine
- Chloroacetamide
- Chlorocresol
- Chloroquinaldol
- Diazolidinyl urea
- Dibromodicyanobutane (phenoxyethanol)
- Dichlorophen
- DMDM hydantoin
- Formaldehyde
- Glutaraldehyde
- Imidazolidinyl urea
- Kathon CG
- Parabens
- Phenylmercuric acetate
- Quaternium-15
- Sorbic acid
- Thimerosal
- Triclosan

### Due to stimulating skin pigmentation:

- *Achillea millefolium* (yarrow)
- *Cananga odorata* (ylang-ylang)
- Dandelion
- Geranium
- Jasmine
- Lavender
- Lemongrass
- Lemon oil
- Neroli
- Peppermint
- Rose oil (Bulgarian)
- Rosemary
- Sandalwood
- Tea tree oil

## Sun Protection for Your Skin

To prevent dark spots and dryness, wear sunscreen regularly. Since sunscreen products can cause redness and irritation and each person reacts to different ingredients, you may have to try several of my recommended products (chosen to minimize skin reaction) before you find one that works for you. Make sure that your combined use of moisturizer, sunscreen, and foundation provides you with a minimum SPF of 15 for daily use.

## RECOMMENDED SUN PROTECTION PRODUCTS

$   Specific Beauty Daily Hydrating Lotion SPF 30
$   Neutrogena Visibly Even Daily Moisturizer SPF 30
$$  Glycolix Elite Sunscreen SPF 30 by Topix
$$  Clarins UV Plus Day Screen SPF 40
$$  La Roche-Posay Ultra Light Fluid SPF 60
$$  Estée Lauder Daywear Plus Multi-Protection Tinted Moisturizer SPF 15
$$  Elta MD UV Clear SPF 46
$$$ SkinCeuticals Ultimate UV Defense SPF 30

**Baumann's Choice:** Neutrogena Visibly Even Daily Moisturizer SPF 30 because it contains essential soy to even skin tone

## Your Makeup

DSPTs often become irritated by ingredients in makeup, but may not recognize that their cosmetics are the source of the problem. DSPTs with an Asian background are especially prone to develop darkness of the skin resulting from a reaction to cosmetic products. Experts believe that this problem, called pigmented contact dermatitis, is induced by very small amounts of allergens that come into almost daily contact with the patient's skin. Eye shadows and blushes are frequent culprits.

If you tend to have darkness on the eyelids, under the eyes, or on the cheeks, consider eliminating cosmetic products that contain ingredients listed previously under "Skin Care Ingredients to Avoid."

You may also find that eye makeup remover can irritate your eyelids, leading to redness and then dark pigmentation. If you suspect that this is your problem, use mineral oil, Vaseline petroleum jelly, or Toleriane Eye Make-Up Remover by La Roche-Posay to remove eye makeup.

Choose foundations containing oil and avoid those labeled oil-free. With your dry skin, you should not be using face powders. And if your skin is very dry, use cream eyeshadows and blushes.

## RECOMMENDED FOUNDATIONS

$  Revlon Colorstay for Normal/Dry Skin Makeup with SoftFlex SPF 15
$  Neutrogena Healthy Skin liquid makeup SPF 20

    $   Jane Iredale PurePressed Base
    $$  Chantecaille Real Skin Foundation
    $$  Laura Mercier Moisturizing Foundation
    $$  M·A·C Studio Fix Fluid Foundation SPF 15
    $$$  Laura Geller Balance-n-Brighten Compact .32 oz

**Baumann's Choice:** Chantecaille Real Skin Foundation

## PROCEDURES FOR YOUR SKIN TYPE

Although your dermatologist can help treat acne, facial flushing, and dark spots, no skin care procedures currently available can improve your skin's dryness and sensitivity. Avoid facials, since they will most likely expose your skin to irritating agents. You may, however, benefit from chemical peels or microdermabrasion to improve dark spots.

## Chemical Peels

Your prescription medication will show results faster if you combine it with dermatologically administered chemical peels. Prescription retinoids enhance the penetration of the peel and will help you heal faster afterward by speeding up cell division. I always advise DSPTs to go to a dermatologist for the peels rather than having them at a spa or salon because your pigmented skin is at risk for developing dark spots with any potentially irritating treatment.

There are many different chemical peel preparations on the market and it is important that you be given the proper one to prevent skin irritation and resulting pigmentation. If you have dark skin or are of Asian ancestry, make sure you see a dermatologist who specializes in skin of color.

## Microdermabrasion

If your S/R score is low (below 40) and you suffer from dark spots on your face, you may benefit from combining microdermabrasion with your depigmenting agent. In microdermabrasion, the practitioner uses a device that sprays microcrystals to remove the upper surface layer of the skin, making it easier for the depigmenting ingredients to penetrate.

If the microdermabrasion is too strong, however, your skin will become inflamed, producing more pigment and worsening your condition. So it's important that you see a dermatologist for these procedures.

## Ongoing Care for Your Type

Fighting dry, sensitive skin will be a lifelong challenge. But putting the proper dietary and skin care routines in place will help. So remember to decrease sun exposure, get enough sleep, avoid irritating products and ingredients, increase humidity in your environment, and use skin care with barrier repair ingredients. Hydrate, hydrate, hydrate.

# CHAPTER FOURTEEN

# Dry, Sensitive, Non-Pigmented, and Wrinkled: DSNW

## ABOUT YOUR SKIN

Relax, DSNW, you *can* manage your reactive skin although, admittedly, yours is not an easy Skin Type.

There's no predicting your skin condition. One day you're fine, and the next, inexplicably, you're having a bad skin day—just when you have that big meeting or date. It's hard to plan and feel confident when you have changeable skin. Dry, flaking, dull, itching, and reddened, often your skin feels uncomfortable and looks irritated. You're puzzled because your desert-dry skin craves moisture, but many products you try cause itching, stinging, and burning. Skin dryness makes wrinkles look worse. If you're in your thirties or older, you may imagine you can see your skin aging day by day. Although moisturizers can help by plumping out fine lines, your sensitive skin won't tolerate most products, even ones designed for sensitive skin.

Antiaging creams are often irritating. When you try a retinoid, your skin may not tolerate the redness and flaking that develop. You're in a double bind: You wrinkle if you don't moisturize, and react if you do. I can identify because I'm on the borderline of DSNT and DSNW, so I treat my skin as a DSNW; so never fear, I know what will work for you.

The good news is that the proper skin care regimen with the right products and ingredients can make a huge difference. In fact, daily skin care is key to addressing your problems. With the right regimen, your skin condition will stabilize, and I'll provide several options to assure that you can care for your skin whatever your particular problem.

## SKIN SENSITIVITY AND THE DSNW

Sensitivity contributes to such skin issues as product and ingredient allergies, rosacea, acne, as well as burning and stinging in response to various substances. Learning to manage your skin's reactivity is a challenge, but understanding why it's occurring can help.

Your key problems result from a damaged skin barrier. The barrier, the outer layer of your skin, is your body's boundary between you and the world. When that boundary is overly permeable, you cannot keep *inside the barrier* important things that you need (such as moisture), and you cannot keep *outside the barrier* problematic things (such as irritants, allergens, and bacteria). Once the skin barrier is damaged, a cycle begins. Lack of protection leads to invasion of substances that cause inflammation; inflammation leads to itching and further breakdown of the protective barrier. As a result, the skin cannot hold on to water, and dehydration results. Dehydration then triggers further inflammation, itching, and dryness.

A whole host of insults can initiate or worsen the barrier breakdown. Preservatives, perfumes, detergents, and other chemicals in skin care products can cause inflammation and damage cells. Ingredients in shampoos, conditioners, hair dyes, shaving products, toners, and soaps can be a problem. Dry-cleaning fluids, chemicals in building materials, carpets, furniture finishes, and industrial and auto pollutants can potentially cause problems in individuals who are allergic.

An allergy patch test performed by a dermatologist or allergist can identify your specific triggers, but the first step is addressing the symptoms by avoiding sensitizing ingredients and using helpful ones. Once the reactive cycle begins, all substances you use must soothe and desensitize. Otherwise, they may further damage your skin barrier and increase your overall skin sensitivity. Later, in the product recommendations section of this chapter, I'll enumerate what to look out for and avoid. If avoiding the most common sensitizers does not produce results, it's advisable to keep a food and product diary, which will help narrow the field if you eventually decide to test for allergies.

## A CLOSE-UP LOOK AT YOUR SKIN

With DSNW skin, you may experience any of the following:

- Dryness
- Scaling and flaking
- Redness
- Burning or stinging

- Wrinkles
- Makeup cakes in wrinkles
- Eye shadows look flaky
- Dry lips with flaking skin
- Rough skin on face
- Lack of skin radiance
- Irritated skin when coming into contact with wool and other rough fabrics
- Mild acne
- Broken blood vessels on face

Most DSNWs are Caucasians from a northern European background. The majority have light skin, which shows every blood vessel, making facial flushing and redness much more obvious. Though annoying, redness is a secondary problem, while dryness, crepiness, and wrinkles are primary skin issues.

## DSNW: A COMPLEX SKIN TYPE

Because DSNW is one of the two most complex Skin Types (the other is DSPW), DSNWs may manifest a variety of different skin problems. Some DSNWs may have few issues—or none. Some may be troubled by one major problem. And some may have the entire range of possible skin problems. It all depends on how you score in each of the four factors measured on the questionnaire. For example, skin sensitivity can result in acne, rosacea, and eczema. If you score high on the sensitivity scale, with a score over 34, you are more likely to have one, two—or all of these three conditions. On the other hand, if your skin is only slightly sensitive, with a score of 24 or less, you may have none of these conditions.

Your O/D score interacts with your S/R score to produce the problems your skin expresses. You may have very dry skin (with a score between 11 and 15), slightly dry skin (with a score between 15 and 18), or combination skin (with a score between 18 and 26). If your skin is combination, your skin sensitivity is more likely to express as acne than as eczema. If your skin is very dry, you are far less likely to get acne, but are more prone to eczema. And once again, if your skin is very sensitive, you could potentially have eczema, acne, and rosacea.

Treating the acne that some (but not all) DSNWs experience can be problematic. Many anti-acne ingredients, such as salicylic acid, benzoyl peroxide, retinol, retinoid, and glycolic acid, are drying. Your over-the-counter treatment options are very limited. Fortunately, a few things I'll recommend later in this chapter can help. Because of your type's complexity, I'll offer a greater range of skin care regimens than I have for most other types. Choose the one right for you, depending upon your skin care needs.

## ROSACEA

Rosacea can be a problem for sensitive, non-pigmented types. To find out if you have any of its symptoms, please consult "The R-Word, Rosacea" in Chapter Six. If you experience any of the rosacea symptoms detailed in Chapter Six, seek help from a dermatologist sooner rather than later because receiving treatment can prevent rosacea from developing to its later stages.

In treating rosacea, several over-the-counter products marketed as "redness relief" contain hydrocortisone or other steroids. Steroids are temporarily effective in shrinking the blood vessels to control redness and calm irritation, but they create a boomerang effect, as blood vessels rebound and enlarge further, worsening the problem. I don't recommend steroid use for that reason. Recently, a friend of my mother's used an "anti-redness" moisturizer; in a week, she developed a beet red face and dermatitis. After a complete review of her skin care regimen, I recognized that the problem was caused by the steroid-containing cream. The tipoff? When she stopped using it, the redness would get worse; when she resumed its use, the redness would stop. This is the "rebound" reaction that occurs with steroid use, creating a dependency on the product. I weaned her from this vicious cycle by introducing a moisturizer with soothing ingredients, like aloe and licorice extract.

## DRY SKIN, DRY ENVIRONMENTS

Dry, sensitive skin can be reactive to ingredients, environmental conditions, fabrics, and stress. Summer can be a challenge because sun exposure worsens redness, dryness, and aging. Your skin doesn't love fall or winter either: blustery winds; parched climates; cold weather; overheated homes, offices, and cars all worsen dry skin. I come from Lubbock, Texas, and its ultradry climate was the bane of my dry, sensitive skin. Who knows? That may be why I learned all about skin care ingredients: to treat *my* skin.

After an airplane flight, during the winter, or in low-humidity environments, your skin will often appear even more dry and wrinkled. When fun-loving friends want to head out onto the slopes for a ski trip, you'd rather stay home or in the nearby ski lodge. Scaling icy peaks is not for you. You'd have to carry your body weight in moisturizers— and even that wouldn't help. Your lips chap, your heels crack. Your face turns red and peels after exposure to icy winds. You try heavy-duty moisturizers, and either they aren't powerful enough or they cause a reaction.

## DSNWs AND AGING PREVENTION

I counsel strict sun avoidance for everyone, even those who tan well, because harmful sun rays accelerate aging and worsen skin conditions like pigmentation and rosacea. However, if I had to single out a type for whom sun exposure produces the most aging effects, it would probably be you. Your non-pigmented skin may have less melanin to handle sun exposure and that's why you burn in the sun. Plus, sun exposure increases rosacea and makes dry skin even drier. Worst of all, your sensitive skin reacts to many sunscreens, causing you to bypass sunscreen—and the end result is premature aging and wrinkling. It's entirely likely that a few bad episodes of burning, along with other genetic and lifestyle factors, have resulted in your scoring as a Wrinkled Type on the questionnaire. So you know what to do: Use sunscreen at all times, indoors and out, and use higher SPFs (45 or above) when you receive direct sun exposure. The products I'll recommend should not cause irritation.

Some DSNWs suffer from acne and/or eczema, and sun exposure is often recommended for these conditions. Although acne was long thought to be "dried out" by the sun, many studies show that acne actually worsens in hot weather. So don't sunbathe to treat your acne.

In some people, eczema arises from an underlying autoimmune condition in which the protective immune system overreacts and attacks itself. Sun exposure temporarily suppresses the immune response, which can lead to a lessening of symptoms for some, but not all, eczema sufferers. Still, since sun exposure contributes to skin aging, why mess around?

DSNWs don't tan well, so my advice is: Give it up. Use strong sun protection, and use it consistently; it's your key step to prevent aging. If you want to tan, use a self-tanner. For more on self-tanners and how to apply them, please refer to "Self-Tanners" in Chapter Ten.

If you needed yet another reason to quit smoking, researchers found that cigarette smoke stimulated an *increased breakdown* of collagen, while lowering collagen production by as much as 40 percent. The more concentrated the smoke, the worse the impact on the skin's collagen. Quit now and your skin will thank you.

## HOW YOUR SKIN TYPE AGES

DSNW skin does not age well, overall. People who experience acne in youth find relief in midlife. But facial flushing, redness, visible veins, sensitivity to skin care products, dryness, and wrinkling are all conditions that worsen with age. People who've failed to follow preventive skin care before their forties feel it now.

Luckily new advances in skin care such as dermal fillers and Botox can address your wrinkles. Advanced skin care products will help treat your skin dryness. Whatever your skin's current condition, it's never too late to take care of your skin.

For postmenopausal women, as estrogen levels go down, you may notice that your skin becomes thinner, drier, and more wrinkled if you do not take hormone replacement therapy. If you wish to consider HRT, first discuss its use with your physician, especially if you or someone in your family has a history of breast cancer or endometrial cancer. Luckily there are some naturally occurring phytoestrogens that can help. Adding phytoestrogen supplements or foods to your diet can be beneficial.

## MOISTURIZING

Moisturize at least twice daily, and don't hesitate to apply creams more often, especially in winter or in low-humidity environments. Because of your skin's tendency to wrinkle, you may be tempted by certain face creams claiming to produce the same results as Botox. These claims are based on the action of skin peptides that in the lab relax muscle cells (or are believed to relax skin cells). Although some research indicates that muscle cells can "relax" in lab settings, it's hard to re-create that same effect outside of the lab. A substance would need to penetrate the epidermis, the dermis, and the fat layer to get to the muscle layer. I've not seen convincing evidence that that can happen. If it could, diabetics could apply their insulin topically rather than injecting it because insulin is a protein, which is composed of peptides. Nor am I convinced that skin cells can "relax," or that it would be beneficial.

Why pay $80 or more for a jar of cream? Many who do may be DSNWs or DRNWs, with dry, wrinkled skin that any moisturizer can improve—temporarily. However, I've yet to see a cream that will deliver the same benefits as Botox. So if you think you need Botox, get Botox. It costs about $300 to $600 per treatment and although its effects are also temporary, it lasts four to six months.

**Dr. Baumann's Bottom Line:** Rebuild your skin barrier and moisturize, avoid harsh ingredients, and protect against drying environments.

## EVERYDAY CARE FOR YOUR SKIN

The goal of your skin care routine is to address skin dryness, wrinkles, and sensitivity (resulting in stinging and redness) with products that deliver hydrating, moisturizing ingredients that do not irritate your skin.

In addition I'll offer an approach to preventing and treating acne, for those of you with acne symptoms.

To address your type's different issues, I've provided two regimens. My first protocol is a hydrating maintenance regimen that may also help acne. Studies show that in many cases, moisturizing the skin will improve acne, even without acne medications, so this regimen concentrates on moisturizing.

The second regimen is designed for those of you who frequently experience redness and stinging in response to skin care products. It uses products with anti-inflammatory and antioxidant ingredients to help rebuild the skin barrier and prevent wrinkles.

If hydrating your skin does not resolve acne, please consult a dermatologist, who can prescribe antibiotics. Your doctor can also recommend an anti-inflammatory medication that treats redness and stinging.

DAILY SKIN CARE

---

### HYDRATING REGIMEN FOR
### MAINTENANCE (AND FOR ACNE):

| AM | PM |
|---|---|
| Step 1: Wash with a cold cream or oil cleanser | Step 1: Wash with a cold cream or oil cleanser |
| Step 2: Apply a moisturizer with SPF and/or sunscreen | Step 2: Apply antioxidant-containing night cream |
| Step 3: Apply a foundation with sunscreen (optional) | Step 3: Once or twice a week use a sulfur-containing mask |

---

In the morning, wash your face with a cold cream or oil cleanser. Apply a moisturizer containing SPF; then, if you wish, apply a foundation with sunscreen. If your skin feels a little oily after using these products, that's all right. You need the protection. Although I don't consider it essential, you can elect to use an eye cream as well, applying it before your moisturizer. In general, I try to avoid exposing your skin to products that are not of real benefit, but if your skin isn't irritated, you can opt to use one.

In the evening, wash with a cold cream or oil cleanser, then apply a night cream that contains antioxidants. Once or twice a week, finish with a mask containing sulfur.

If hydrating your skin with this regimen does not improve your acne, you need to see a dermatologist. Unfortunately, the over-the-counter ingredients available to treat acne will dry your skin out. DSNWs do well with a prescription topical antibiotic or light treatments (see "Procedures," later in chapter) to treat acne.

## REGIMEN FOR FACIAL REDNESS
## OR FREQUENT STINGING:

| AM | PM |
|---|---|
| Step 1: Wash with a cream or oil cleanser | Step 1: Wash with a cream or oil cleanser |
| Step 2: Rinse with facial water | Step 2: Rinse with facial water |
| Step 3: Apply anti-inflammatory serum or lotion | Step 3: Apply an antioxidant and/or anti-inflammatory night cream |
| Step 4: Apply a moisturizer with SPF and/or sunscreen | Step 4: Once or twice a week, use a hydrating mask with antioxidant and/or anti-inflammatory ingredients |
| Step 5: Apply a foundation with sunscreen (optional) | |

In the morning, wash your face with a cream or oil cleanser, then rinse with facial water, not tap water. Next, apply a moisturizer containing SPF, and finish with a foundation containing sunscreen. I do not recommend eye cream when your skin is reddened and reactive.

In the evening, wash with a cream or oil cleanser, and rinse your face using facial water. Apply a night cream that contains antioxidant and/or anti-inflammatory ingredients (see the lists that follow for product and ingredient recommendations).

Once or twice a week, use a hydrating mask that also contains antioxidant and/or anti-inflammatory ingredients.

## Cleansers

As a DSNW, you need gentle, hydrating cleansers. To use, apply a small amount to your face with a soft, clean washcloth, using gentle circular motions over your entire face. To rinse, spray facial water over your face and tissue off whatever cleanser remains. If your skin is only slightly sensitive, you can rinse with regular tap water.

## RECOMMENDED CLEANSING PRODUCTS

$ CeraVe Hydrating Cleanser

$ Burt's Bees Soap Bark & Chamomile Deep Cleansing Cream Soap Bark & Chamomile

$ Eucerin Redness Relief Soothing Cleanser

$ Cetaphil Skin Cleanser

$$ Nia24 Gentle Cleanser

$$ La Roche-Posay Toleriane Dermo-Cleanser

$$ Biotherm Biosource Softening Cleansing Milk for Dry Skin

$$ VMV Moisture Rich Creammmy Cleansing Milk

$$ Shu Uemura High Performance Balancing Cleansing Oil Advanced Formula

$$ Vivite Hydrating Facial Cleanser

$$$ Darphin Intral Cleansing Milk

$$$ Caudalie Gentle Cleanser

$$$ La Prairie Purifying Cream Cleanser

**Baumann's Choice:** If you have frequent redness and stinging, use Toleriane Dermo-Cleanser by La Roche-Posay. I personally use the Vivite Hydrating Facial Cleanser.

## Facial Waters

DSNWs should never use toners, which are drying. Instead, use these special facial waters either to remove cleansers or to spray on the face after cleansing, before applying moisturizer. Water, especially hot hard water, has been shown to irritate the skin. For skin that is not raw and sensitive, you can use tap water but make sure it's lukewarm.

### RECOMMENDED FACIAL WATERS

$ Evian Mineral Water Spray

$ Vichy Thermal Spa Water

$$ Avène Thermal Water Spray

$$ Chantecaille Pure Rosewater

$$ Fresh Rose Marigold Tonic Water

$$ Jurlique Chamomile Soothing Mist

$$ La Roche-Posay Thermal Spring Water

$$ Shu Uemura Depsea Hydrability Moisturizing Emulsion

**Baumann's Choice:** La Roche-Posay Thermal Spring Water

## Serums

Anti-inflammatory serums and lotions contain powerful ingredients to help calm sensitivity. Use them before you apply a daytime moisturizer with SPF.

### RECOMMENDED ANTI-INFLAMMATORY SERUMS AND LOTIONS

- $ Aveeno Ultra-Calming Daily Moisturizer SPF 15
- $ Josie Maran Argan Oil
- $ Paula's Choice Resist Super Antioxidant Concentrate Serum
- $$ Replenix Power of 3 Cream
- $$ La Roche-Posay Rosaliac Perfecting Anti-Redness Moisturizer
- $$ SoPhyto Multivitamin Skin Drops
- $$$ iS Clinical Pro-Heal Serum Advance (Not for those with stinging skin)
- $$$ Combray by Solenne

**Baumann's Choice:** Aveeno Ultra-Calming Daily Moisturizer because it contains feverfew

## Moisturizers

Sensitive skin needs to be moisturized at least twice a day. When your skin is especially dry, moisturize more often. For daytime use, I've included products with antioxidant and anti-inflammatory ingredients. Use a product with SPF.

### RECOMMENDED DAYTIME MOISTURIZERS

- $ Eucerin Sensitive Facial Skin $Q_{10}$ Anti-Wrinkle Sensitive Skin Lotion SPF 15
- $ Aveeno Positively Ageless Lifting & Firming Moisturizer SPF 30
- $ Purpose Dual Treatment Moisture Lotion with SPF 15
- $$ La Roche-Posay Hydraphase UV SPF 30
- $$ Canyon Ranch Your Transformation Protect UVA/UVB
- $$ Clinique Comfort On Call Allergy Tested Relief Cream
- $$ L'Occitane Ultra Moisturizing Fluid SPF 20

$$ Vichy UV Active Daily Moisturizer Cream with Sunscreen SPF 15

$$$ Bobbi Brown Extra SPF 25 Moisturizing Balm

**Baumann's Choice:** L'Occitane Ultra Moisturizing Fluid SPF 20

### RECOMMENDED EVENING MOISTURIZERS

$ Eucerin Sensitive Facial Cream Skin $Q_{10}$ Anti-Wrinkle Sensitive

$ Aveeno Positively Ageless Night Cream

$$ Alchimie Forever Kantic + Intensely Nourishing Cream

$$ Atopalm MLE Cream

$$ Vivite Replenish Hydrating Cream

$$ SK-II Skin Signature Melting Rich Cream (If you prefer heavy creams)

$$$ Kinerase Pro+Therapy Ultra Rich Night Repair (Do not use when irritated)

$$ La Roche-Posay Toleriane Soothing Protective Facial Cream

$$ Biotherm Nutrisource Ultra Comforting Rich Cream

$$ Nia24 Intensive Recovery Complex

$$$ Fresh Creme Ancienne (If you like heavy creams)

$$$ Caudalie Premier Cru

**Baumann's Choice:** Atopalm MLE Cream with pseudoceramides that help build the skin barrier. Great to use when skin is red, sore, and irritated.

## Masks

Masks can be very helpful for DSNWs; a sulfur mask will help reduce inflammation and acne, while hydrating masks help repair the skin barrier.

My favorite mask for improving acne is actually a prescription product: Plexion SCT mask by Medicis, which contains sulfacetamide to help reduce inflammation. It's worth a visit to your dermatologist.

### RECOMMENDED MASKS FOR ACNE SUFFERERS

$$ DDF Sulfur Therapeutic Mask

$$ Peter Thomas Roth Sulfur Cooling Masque

**Baumann's Choice:** DDF Sulfur Therapeutic Mask

## RECOMMENDED MASKS TO HYDRATE SKIN

$   MD Formulations Moisture Defense Treatment Masque
$$   Alchimie Forever Kantic Mask
$$   Kate Somerville Quench Hydrating Mask
$$   Caudalie Vinosource Moisturizing Cream-Mask
$$   Elizabeth Arden Hydrating Mask
$$   Fresh Rose Face Mask

**Baumann's Choice:** Kate Somerville Quench Hydrating Mask because it contains soothing ingredients such as willow herb and cucumber

## SHOPPING FOR PRODUCTS

Look for products containing ingredients that will effectively hydrate and protect your skin. Avoid products that will irritate your sensitive skin. I can't list all detergents to avoid because much depends on their concentrations and formulations, so the easiest guideline is to avoid any products—be they cleansers, shampoos, or bubble baths—that foam. If you feel you must use a foaming cleanser, make sure it has minimal rather than thick foam. You should also avoid fragrances, which can lead to skin allergy.

On the following pages, I've listed other ingredients to avoid. If you have a favorite skin care product that is not on my recommended list, please go to www.skintypesolutions.com and tell me what it is. I am always looking for the next new thing!

---

### RECOMMENDED SKIN CARE INGREDIENTS

#### *For wrinkle prevention:*

- Basil
- Caffeine
- *Camilla sinensis* (green tea, white tea)
- Carrot extract
- Coenzyme $Q_{10}$ (ubiquinone)
- Copper peptide
- Curcumin (tetrahydracurcumin or turmeric)
- Ferulic acid
- Ginseng
- Grape seed extract
- Idebenone
- Lutein
- Lycopene
- *Punica granatum* (pomegranate)
- Pycnogenol (a pine bark extract)
- Rosemary

- Feverfew
- Genistein (soy)
- Ginger
- Silymarin
- Yucca

## To improve wrinkles:

- Copper peptide
- *Ginkgo biloba*

## Anti-inflammatory:

- Aloe vera
- Chamomile
- Colloidal oatmeal
- Cucumber
- Dexpanthenol (pro-vitamin $B_5$)
- *Epilobium angustifolium* (willow herb)
- Evening primrose oil
- Feverfew
- Green tea
- Licochalone
- Perilla leaf extract
- Pycnogenol (a pine bark extract)
- Red algae
- Thyme
- *Trifolium pretense* (red clover)
- Zinc

## For moisturizing:

- *Ajuga turkestanica*
- Aloe vera
- Apricot kernel oil
- Borage seed oil
- Canola oil
- Ceramide
- Cholesterol
- Cocoa butter (not if you have acne)
- Colloidal oatmeal
- Dexpanthenol (pro-vitamin $B_5$)
- Dimethicone
- Evening primrose oil
- Glycerin
- Jojoba oil
- Macadamia nut oil
- Olive oil
- Safflower oil
- Shea butter

### SKIN CARE INGREDIENTS TO AVOID

## If you have acne:

- Butyl stearate
- Cinnamon oil
- Isostearyl palmitate
- Lanolin

- Cocoa butter
- Coconut oil
- Decyl oleate
- Isocetyl stearate
- Isopropyl isostearate
- Isopropyl myristate
- Isopropyl neopentanoate
- Myristyl myristate
- Myristyl propionate
- Octyl palmitate
- Octyl stearate
- Peppermint oil
- Propylene glycol-2 (PPG-2)

### *If you have skin redness:*

- Alpha hydroxy acids (lactic acid, glycolic acid)
- Alpha lipoic acid
- Benzoyl peroxide
- Gluconolactone
- Phytic acid
- Polyhydroxy acids
- Retinaldehyde
- Retinol
- Retinyl palmitate
- Salicylic acid (beta hydroxy acid)
- Vitamin C (l-ascorbic acid)

### *Due to allergy or irritation:*

- Bismuth oxychloride (found in eye shadow)
- Castor oil and eosin (both found in long-lasting lipsticks)
- Chromium hydroxide and chromium oxide compounds (give makeup the green color but can cause allergy)
- Cobalt
- Lead
- Nickel
- Propyl gallate
- Ricinoleic acid

## Sun Protection for Your Skin

Use cream sunscreens to give your skin extra moisture. If you react to chemical sunscreen ingredients like avobenzone and benzophenone with redness and sensitivity, look for sunscreens containing dimethicone and cyclomethicone, which may prevent irritation from other sunscreen ingredients in those with easily irritated skin.

## RECOMMENDED SUN PROTECTION PRODUCTS

$   Neutrogena Sensitive Skin Sunblock Lotion with SPF 30
$$   Citrix Antioxidant Sunscreen SPF 30
$$   Aveeno Ultra-Calming Moisturizing Lotion with SPF 30
$$   Origins Sunshine State SPF 20
$$   Philosophy The Supernatural Poreless, Flawless SPF 15
$$   SkinCeuticals Physical UV Defense SPF 30
$$$   Darphin Vital Protection Age-Defying Protective Lotion SPF 50

**Baumann's Choice:** Aveeno Ultra-Calming Moisturizing Lotion with SPF 30

---

### SUNSCREEN INGREDIENTS TO SUSPECT IF REDNESS OR STINGING OCCURS

- Avobenzone (Parsol)
- Benzophenone
- Methoxycinnamate
- Para-aminobenzoic acid (PABA)

---

## Your Makeup

Your dry, sensitive skin is likely to react with redness to allergens in makeup. While foundations are usually not a problem, blushes and eye shadow can be.

Many brands of eye shadow contain lead, cobalt, nickel, and chromium, ingredients that can cause allergy in susceptible people. Shimmery shadows, blushes, and bronzers may contain sharp-edged particles like shells that can scratch and irritate dry, sensitive skin, as well as make the wrinkles look more prominent.

Cream eye shadows and blushes are best, but if your cheeks are naturally pink, you can skip the blush. (I do.) Powders, usually designed for oil control, are unnecessary and may make skin appear drier and more wrinkled. If you want coverage without using a heavy foundation, use tinted moisturizers with sunscreen. For very dry skin, apply it *over* your moisturizer. If your skin is only slightly dry, use the moisturizer on its own.

Foundations containing salicylic acid (BHA) to help improve acne are too drying for you. Stick to oil-containing foundations. Oil, contrary to popular belief, will not increase acne breakouts.

## RECOMMENDED FOUNDATIONS

$ Revlon Age Defying Makeup with Botafirm
$$ Kevyn Aucoin The Dew Drop Foundation
$$ Jane Iredale Dream Tint SPF 15
$$ Trish McEvoy Protective Shield Tinted Moisturizer
$$$ La Prairie Skin Caviar Concealer Foundation SPF 15
$$$ M·A·C Studio Fix Fluid Foundation SPF 15

**Baumann's Choice:** Revlon Age Defying Makeup with Botafirm

## RECOMMENDED CREAM EYE SHADOWS

$ Almay Bright Eyes
$ Revlon Illuminance Creme Shadow
$$ Bliss Lidthicks
$$ Bobbi Brown Cream Shadow Stick
$$ Clinique Touch Tint for Eyes Cream Formula

**Baumann's Choice:** Bliss Lidthicks with antioxidants

## RECOMMENDED BLUSHES

$ Avon Split Second Blush Stick
$ Mary Kay MK Signature Cheek Color
$ Revlon Cream Blush
$$ Bobbi Brown Cream Blush Stick
$$ Jane Iredale Blush (powder blush with soothing minerals)
$$ h.wood.lips Shine Pots (for lips and cheeks)

**Baumann's Choice:** If you purchase the h.wood.lips product, don't miss their Lip Tea Scrubs, which are edible lip exfoliators.

## PROCEDURES FOR YOUR SKIN TYPE

Unfortunately there are no skin care procedures that can improve your dry, sensitive skin. If you suffer from frequent skin rashes in reaction to cosmetic products, your dermatologist can help you figure out what ingredients in these products are causing your rash by performing a series of patch tests. (See Chapter Fifteen, "Procedures for Your Skin Type," for information on patch testing.)

## Treatments for Wrinkles

Although using the right moisturizer can improve some of your fine wrinkles, for the rest of them you may want to consider using botulinum toxin or dermal fillers.

## Light Treatments

Certain forms of light treatments, light emitting diodes, and Intense Pulsed Light will probably be used in the future to prevent or treat wrinkles. Right now, though, the technology is not that effective for wrinkle treatment, though fine for other purposes. (I've seen people who've spent $5,000 to $6,000 on these treatments without seeing improvement in their wrinkles.) Several lasers such as the Fraxel and Titan have been effective on wrinkles.

However, light treatments *are* effective in treating some symptoms of rosacea and acne.

## What About Chemical Peels?

If redness and stinging is your problem, you don't need chemical peels, which contain ingredients that may make your skin more red and sensitive. Due to your impaired skin barrier, you can be burned by a vigorous peel. Stay away from these procedures. However, if you have acne without redness or stinging, you may benefit from chemical peels. My favorite chemical peel ingredients for acne are salicylic acid (BHA) and resorcinol.

## ONGOING CARE FOR YOUR SKIN TYPE

Choose your products with care and moisturize regularly. Avoid the sun, quit smoking, and don't forget to eat your vegetables.

# CHAPTER FIFTEEN

# Dry, Sensitive, Non-Pigmented, and Tight: DSNT

## BAUMANN SKIN TYPE NUMBER 2

■

*"I do not have any aging issues yet but my dry sensitive skin drives me crazy—especially in the winter. I am not sure why my skin is so sensitive and would like to try and crack the code."*

## ABOUT YOUR SKIN

Scaling, flaking, reddened, rough, and dull. If your questionnaire results show you to be a DSNT, your skin is literally thirsting for water. It's like that famous line from *The Rime of the Ancient Mariner:* "Water, water, everywhere, nor any drop to drink." You've tried everything. You followed the advice to keep well hydrated by consuming quarts of water per day, to no avail. You avoid caffeine because of its dehydrating effects. You know you need to moisturize, and in desperation, you try every product that comes along—but even the most costly creams can cause reactions in your sensitive skin.

Understanding your skin is the basis for making the right skin care choices. I am on the cusp between a DSNW and DSNT. It isn't the easiest, and at least one of the reasons I've become so passionate about ingredients and products was to learn how to address my *own* skin challenges. So never fear, there is a Skin Type solution even for your fragile, dry skin.

## OVERVIEW OF DSNT SKIN

Fair-skinned Caucasians who take good care of themselves and their skin most commonly have this type. Although its delicacy is much admired, caring for it can be a pain. You don't tan well. You'd do best to avoid the sun completely. Most DSNTs have figured out that excess sun is not a friend to supersensitive dry skin. Those who have not figured that out are paying the price, and it's likely that they would fall into the DSNW Skin Type, which is similar but wrinkled. At least you don't have to deal with preventing and addressing wrinkles. "Aren't wrinkles inevitable?" many people wonder. No, they are not. Skin that never sees the sun does not wrinkle, so with the right behaviors wrinkles can be avoided, although the loss of fat in the face that occurs with aging cannot. Tight-skinned DSNs can congratulate themselves on good habits, like sun avoidance and smoking cessation. Many DSNTs also eat a healthy diet full of antioxidants (obtained from fruits and vegetables), which helps prevent wrinkles and maintain overall health.

Still, keeping your skin calm, hydrated, and nonreactive at any age takes some work, along with careful product selection.

## SKIN SENSITIVITY AND THE DSNT

Forty percent of Americans report that they have sensitive skin that reacts to products and ingredients with burning, stinging, itching, and redness. Since tracking down the exact culprit can be time-consuming, I recommend that you first eliminate common triggers by avoiding ingredients enumerated later in the product recommendations section of this chapter. If this does not produce results, you can always keep a food and product diary, writing down what you eat and what you use on your skin, so that you can track your reactions to potential allergens and ingredients. Ultimately, you can go to a dermatologist for patch testing, which will determine the precise allergen. But that process is less expensive if you have first narrowed the field.

Skin sensitivities and skin allergies are on the same spectrum; while you may not always be actively allergic to a particular skin care ingredient, unless that substance is soothing and desensitizing, it can also damage your skin barrier and increase your overall skin sensitivity.

## THE SKIN BARRIER

The skin's natural barrier is composed of cells (something like bricks) that are surrounded by fat (called lipids), which acts as mortar. The fat molecules line up in a lipid bilayer (two rows of fat molecules) to form a three-dimensional structure. It functions like Saran Wrap, keeping water inside the layers of the skin, while keeping allergens, toxins, and bacteria out.

With a weak skin barrier, substances pass through the barrier too readily, producing allergic or inflammatory reactions as the immune system recognizes something foreign to the body and overreacts. Once the skin barrier is damaged, a cycle begins. Lack of protection leads to invasion of substances that cause inflammation; inflammation leads to itching and further breakdown of the barrier. As a result, the skin cannot hold on to water, and dehydration results.

A whole host of insults can initiate or worsen the barrier breakdown. Skin care ingredients that are harsh or perfumed can cause inflammation and break down cells. DSNTs fared better when "fragrance free" was the rage. Acetone in nail polish, chemicals used to treat fabric, dry-cleaning fluids, chemicals in building materials, carpets, furniture finishes, and industrial and auto pollutants can potentially cause problems.

Many DSNTs suffer from skin allergies. Many can't wear earrings that are not real gold or platinum, without getting a rash. This is often due to a nickel allergy. Watches and hooks on clothing or undergarments can cause rashes to develop. Red rashes may appear underneath a ring, but don't worry. It's not that your gold or platinum ring is phony. The more likely explanation is that when you wash your hands, soap detergent gets caught under the ring and irritates your skin.

People who come from families with allergies and asthma are more prone to the dryness leading to eczema. This may be due to an abnormality of an enzyme that helps maintain the structure of the skin.

In oily types, skin sensitivity will cause acne and flushing, while stinging, burning, and allergic reactions are less common because oil helps strengthen the skin barrier. However, those with a high score on the Sensitivity vs. Resistance scale will commonly experience allergies to many skin ingredients. Oily/dry combination types with sensitive skin will have more infrequent outbreaks, such as a few pimples every few months. In dry, sensitive types, dryness leading to eczema is the chief concern. The drier and the more sensitive your skin scored on the questionnaire, the higher your risk factor.

With DSNT skin you may experience any of the following:

- Dryness
- Flaking
- Scaling
- Itching
- Blotches
- Redness
- Sensitivity to skin care ingredients
- Sensitivity to soaps and detergents
- Rashes under rings
- Rashes from jewelry that is not real gold or platinum
- Irritation and inflammation from pierced earrings
- Occasional pimples

Dry skin may be more than a skin-deep problem. It may be a symptom of hypothyroidism, a disease that is on the rise. Please consult your doctor to find out if you are at risk.

## ENVIRONMENTAL AGENTS THAT CAN LEAD TO DRY SKIN

If you are experiencing extreme dryness or eczema, notice if any of these conditions could be contributing:

- Cold weather
- Dry climate
- Wind
- Prolonged exposure to hot water
- Detergents and soaps
- Friction from rough clothing
- Frequent air travel
- Air-conditioning
- Pollution

While many of these conditions are unavoidable, you can take protective action such as wearing extra moisturizer, covering your face in cold or windy conditions, and purchasing softer fabrics if you notice a problem.

Airplane travel is a problem for everyone, but Dry Skin Types are the most affected. Whatever the outer conditions, our body's natural mechanisms work to maintain a constant level of water within every cell, and this includes skin cells too. It takes three days for the skin to rebalance after travel. For recommendations on protecting your skin during air travel, please consult page 322.

Soaking in hot water can also dry and potentially damage DSNT skin. Hot baths, steam rooms, and facials are not for you. Instead take a quick shower using moderately warm water. Watch out for water quality. Hard or chemically treated water can be drying. Apply moisturizer after exiting the shower, while you're still damp, to trap residual water on the skin surface. Prolonged immersion (over an hour) in room-temperature water can disrupt the skin barrier.

Shampoos and conditioners that contact your face as you rinse should also be selected with care. Read labels to avoid the most common sensitizing ingredients. Always rinse thoroughly after use. Bubbly shampoos pose the biggest risk, so avoid getting the shampoo on your face.

Even cleansing can further dry out DSNT skin unless you use a specially formulated cleanser. I'll point you toward the best products later in this chapter.

## MOISTURIZERS AND DSNT SKIN

Although your thirsty dry skin desperately needs moisturizer, in my opinion, your needs can be well served by products in the low-to-moderate price range. In most instances, the higher-end moisturizers are unnecessary—unless you can afford them and happen to like their packaging.

Although I recommend the use of retinol- and retinoid-containing products for those with oily or pigmented skin and for those prone to wrinkles, since you have non-pigmented, tight skin, they aren't necessary for you. Plus, despite their antiaging benefits, they can be drying and should be used selectively by only some of the Dry Types.

## REPAIRING YOUR SKIN BARRIER

Now that I've alerted you to the problems caused by a weak barrier and the external conditions that may contribute to barrier damage, here comes the good news: what you can do to rebuild the barrier. Since it's composed of fatty acids, both the types of fats (and oils) that you eat and the types of fats (and oils) that you use on your skin can impact the barrier. Ingesting and using topically the right types of fats (and oils) is thought to be very important to maintain a healthy skin barrier and to repair a damaged one.

The three main components of a well-functioning skin barrier are cholesterol, fatty acids, and ceramides, different types of fat molecules that must be present in the right ratio to form the correct three-dimensional structure to make the skin watertight.

Anything that disrupts any of these three types of fats either internally or externally can therefore undermine the structure of the skin barrier. Taking drugs that lower cholesterol levels worsens dry skin. Detergents, like sodium lauryl sulfate, strip fatty acids, leading to dry skin and irritation, research reveals. Sun exposure inhibits enzymes that help to make ceramides, resulting in dry skin.

While many skin care products contain one or more of the key fats needed for skin repair, the best products contain all three in the right ratio.

In the next section of this chapter, I'll show you how to use the right kinds of products and ingredients to moisturize and rebuild your skin.

**Dr. Baumann's Bottom Line:** Prevent dryness by avoiding the detergents, soaps, harsh chemicals, and other environmental assaults that can undermine the solidity of your skin barrier. It's easier to prevent damage than to treat it once it occurs. Eat right, reduce stress, and take supplements with omega-3 fats. Use moisturizers that contain all three lipids needed to rebuild the barrier: cholesterol, fatty acids, and ceramides. Address dryness, lessen sensitivity, and soothe irritation.

## EVERYDAY CARE FOR YOUR SKIN

The goal of your skin care routine is to make your skin less dry and sensitive, using products that deliver ingredients that repair the skin barrier. In addition, your daily regimen will help to prevent and treat acne.

As a DSNT, your needs are relatively simple. You need to avoid ingredients (such as alcohol) and products (such as foaming cleansers) that strip the necessary natural lipids from your skin. And second, use moisturizers with ingredients that help build and maintain your skin barrier.

Your type has an increased risk of eczema (which usually occurs on the body, not the face). If you suffer from recurring red, dry, itching patches on your skin, see a dermatologist and get prescription medications to treat it.

## DAILY SKIN CARE

### REGIMEN

| AM | PM |
|---|---|
| Step 1: Wash with non-foaming creamy cleanser | Step 1: Wash with non-foaming cleanser |
| Step 2: Apply anti-inflammatory serum | Step 2: Apply anti-inflammatory serum |
| Step 3: Spray soothing facial water | Step 3: Spray soothing facial water |
| Step 4: Apply eye cream (optional) | Step 4: Apply eye cream (optional) |
| Step 5: Immediately apply moisturizer with SPF or combination of moisturizer, sunscreen, and foundation for a total SPF of 15 or more | Step 5: Immediately apply night cream |

In the morning, wash your face with a non-foaming creamy cleanser, then apply an anti-inflammatory serum. Next, spray facial water. Apply an eye cream, if desired, and finish with a moisturizer that contains SPF. Make sure to apply moisturizing products while skin is still moist, to trap water in skin.

In the evening, wash with the same cleanser used in the morning and apply the same anti-inflammatory serum. Spray facial water, apply eye cream if you are using one, and apply a night cream.

Undertake this regimen for two weeks. If your skin does not improve, try another set of recommended products. If there is still no improvement after you have tried three sets of products, see a dermatologist.

## Cleansers

Use only moisturizing, non-foaming cleansers. Never use ordinary soap.

## RECOMMENDED CLEANSERS

- $ Eucerin Redness Relief Soothing Cleanser
- $ Neutrogena Sensitive Skin Solutions Cream Cleanser
- $ Nivea Visage Gentle Cleansing Cream, Dry & Sensitive Skin
- $ Olay Total Effects Nourishing Cream Cleanser
- $ Aveeno Ultra Calming Moisturizing Cream Cleanser
- $$ Vivite Replenish Hydrating Facial Cleanser
- $$ Arbonne NutriMinC RE⁹ Renewing Gelée Crème Hydrating Wash
- $$ Kate Somerville Gentle Daily Wash
- $$ Elemis Rose Petal Cleanser
- $$ La Roche-Posay Toleriane Dermo-Cleanser
- $$ Biotherm Biosource Softening Cleansing Milk for Dry Skin
- $$ VMV Moisture Rich Creammmy Cleansing Milk (for Dry Skin)
- $$$ Christian Dior Prestige Cleansing Crème
- $$$ Shu Uemura High Performance Balancing Cleansing Oil Fresh
- $$$ La Prairie Purifying Cream Cleanser

**Baumann's Choice:** Biotherm Biosource Softening Cleansing Milk for Dry Skin

## Serums

Serums can confer powerful ingredients to help manage the inflammation that occurs with skin sensitivity. Most serums are too irritating for a DS Type, but I can recommend these below.

## RECOMMENDED SERUMS

- $$ Dr. Andrew Weil for Origins Plantidote Mega-Mushroom Face Serum
- $$ Elizabeth Arden Overnight Success-Skin Renewal Serum
- $$ Joey New York Calm and Correct Serum
- $$ La Roche-Posay Toleriane Facial Fluid
- $$ iS Clinical Pro-Heal Serum Advance
- $$$ Combray Serum

**Baumann's Choice:** iS Clinical Pro-Heal Serum Advance is my favorite unless stinging is a concern for you.

## Facial Water

DSNTs should never use toners, which are designed to strip much-needed fats out of the skin and may contain alcohol and other drying ingredients. Instead, use a facial water. You can learn more about the benefits of facial water in Chapter Thirteen, on page 216. Spray the water on your face immediately prior to applying an eye cream and moisturizer. The creams will help trap the water on the skin, giving the skin a reservoir to pull from. This is particularly helpful in low-humidity environments.

### RECOMMENDED FACIAL WATERS

$ Evian Mineral Water Spray

$ Vichy Thermal Spa Water

$$ Arbonne NutriMinC RE⁹ Restoring Mist Balancing Toner

$$ Avene Thermal Spring Water

$$ Chantecaille Pure Rosewater

$$ Fresh Rose Marigold Tonic Water

$$ La Roche-Posay Thermal Spring Water

$$ Shu Uemura Depsea Water Facial Mist (Fragrance Free)

**Baumann's Choice:** La Roche-Posay Thermal Spring Water has selenium, which helps decrease inflammation.

## Moisturizers

DSNTs need to moisturize as much as possible. The correct moisturizers will do more for your skin than anything else. Select different ones for morning and evening because the evening products may be too greasy for daytime, preventing your makeup from spreading well. If you use a daytime moisturizer that contains an SPF of 15, you won't need to apply an additional sunscreen. However, if your moisturizer contains less than that amount, you can use any combination of moisturizer, sunscreen, and foundation with SPF to assure you attain that coverage.

### RECOMMENDED DAYTIME MOISTURIZERS

$ Aveeno Ultra-Calming Daily Moisturizer SPF 15

$ Cetaphil Daily Facial Moisturizer SPF 15

$ Good Skin All Calm Gentle Sunscreen SPF 25

$   Purpose Dual Treatment Moisture Lotion with SPF 15
$$  SkinCeuticals Daily Sun Defense SPF 20
$$  Topix Glycolix Elite Sunscreen SPF 30
$$$ Nia24 Sun Damage Prevention 100% Mineral Sunscreen

**Baumann's Choice:** Aveeno Ultra-Calming Daily Moisturizer SPF 15 because it contains feverfew

### RECOMMENDED EVENING MOISTURIZERS

$   Aveeno Ultra-Calming Moisturizing Cream
$   Yes To Tomatoes Totally Tranquil Facial Hydrating Lotion
$   Eucerin Redness Relief Soothing Night Cream
$$  Atopalm MLE Cream
$$  Burt's Bees Evening Primrose Overnight Crème
$$  Clarins Multi-Active Night Youth Recovery Comfort Cream
$$  Elizabeth Arden Good Night's Sleep Restoring Cream
$$  Jurlique Wrinkle Softener Beauty Cream
$$$ Crème de la Mer
$$$ Sisley Botanical Moisturizer with Cucumber

**Baumann's Choice:** Atopalm MLE Cream

## Eye Creams

Don't feel you have to use a separate eye cream. Using your nighttime moisturizer around the eye area is fine, unless you find it too heavy. Here are some suggestions for those who prefer a separate eye cream.

### RECOMMENDED EYE CREAMS

$   Neutrogena Skin Soothing Eye Tints
$   Olay Definity Eye Treatment
$$  Biotherm Aquasource Biosensitive Eye Contour Hydrator
$$$ Caudalie Vinexpert Anti-Aging Serum Eyes and Lips
$$$ Kinerase Ultra Rich Eye Repair
$$$ Jo Malone Green Tea & Honey Eye Cream
$$$ Lancôme Absolue Eye Premium Bx Absolute Replenishing Eye Cream
$$$ Murad Lighten and Brighten Eye Treatment

**Baumann's Choice:** Olay Definity Highly Defined Anti-Aging Illuminating Eye Treatment because it contains niacinamide

## Exfoliation

DSNTs should not exfoliate unless they have a low S/R score of 30 or below. Those of you with higher S/R scores will likely develop facial redness and increased sensitivity if you try it. However, you can use a very light scrub with an emollient base once a week to help remove dry skin flakes. Just don't overdo it. My favorite product is the Clinique 7 Day Scrub Cream.

## SHOPPING FOR PRODUCTS

Never use soaps—or any products—that contain detergents. How can you tell? First, notice the product's action. Though a small amount of foam is acceptable, if a cleanser, soap, shampoo, or bath product produces vigorous suds and bubbles, it contains detergent. Stay away from it.

Second, read ingredient lists and make sure you avoid all detergents and sensitizing ingredients you find listed on the labels of skin care products and any other products that contact your skin, such as shampoos and other hair products, as well as bath and body products. Sodium lauryl sulfate is an irritating detergent commonly used in shampoos, conditioners, and other skin care products. Look out for it, and purchase brands that *don't* contain it. The lists that follow will alert you to other ingredients you should avoid.

---

**RECOMMENDED SKIN CARE INGREDIENTS**

### *To prevent dark spots:*

- *Cocos nucifera* (coconut extract), unless you have acne
- Cucumber
- Niacinamide
- Pycnogenol (a pine bark extract)
- *Saxifraga sarmentosa* extract (strawberry begonia)
- Soy

## To improve dark spots:

- Arbutin
- Cucumber extract
- *Glycyrrhiza glabra* (licorice extract)

- Hydroquinone

## To prevent inflammation:

- Aloe vera
- Chamomile
- Colloidal oatmeal
- Cucumber
- Dexpanthenol (pro-vitamin B$_5$)
- *Epilobium angustifolium* (willow herb)
- Evening primrose oil

- Feverfew
- Perilla leaf extract
- Pycnogenol (a pine bark extract)
- Red algae
- Thyme
- *Trifolium pretense* (red clover)

## To increase moisture:

- Borage seed oil
- Castor oil
- Ceramide
- Cholesterol
- Cocoa butter (avoid if you have acne)
- Colloidal oatmeal
- Dexpanthenol (pro-vitamin B$_5$)
- Dimethicone

- Evening primrose oil
- Glycerin
- Jojoba oil
- Olive oil
- Pumpkin seed oil
- Safflower oil
- Stearic acid and other fatty acids
- Sunflower oil

### SKIN CARE INGREDIENTS TO AVOID

## Due to irritating detergents:

- Dimethyl dodecyl amido betaine
- Lauryl sulfates

- Sodium dodecyl sulfate
- Sodium lauryl sulfate

### Due to increasing acne or skin redness:

- Cinnamon oil
- Cocoa butter
- *Cocos nucifera* (coconut oil)
- Isopropyl isostearate
- Isopropyl myristate
- Peppermint oil

### Due to problematic preservatives:

- Benzalkonium chloride
- Bronopol
- Chloroacetamide
- Chlorocresol
- Chlorohexidine
- Chloroquinaldol
- Diazolidinyl urea
- Dibromodicyanobutane (phenoxyethanol)
- Dichlorophen
- DMDM hydantoin
- Formaldehyde
- Glutaraldehyde
- Imidazolidinyl urea
- Kathon CG
- Parabens
- Phenylmercuric acetate
- Quaternium-15
- Sorbic acid
- Thimerosal
- Triclosan

## Sun Protection for Your Skin

Although I recommend that you rely upon an SPF-containing moisturizer to keep well protected, you may also wish to reapply sunscreen regularly, choosing any of my selections.

### RECOMMENDED SUNSCREENS

$   Blue Lizard Australian Sunscreen SPF 30+, Sensitive
$   Purpose Dual Treatment Moisturizer SPF 15
$$  La Roche-Posay Anthelios SX SPF 15
$$  SkinCeuticals Daily Sun Defense SPF 20
$$  Topix Pharmaceuticals Glycolix Elite Sunscreen SPF 30

**Baumann's Choice:** La Roche-Posay Anthelios SX SPF 15

| SUNSCREEN INGREDIENTS TO AVOID |
| --- |

*If you get skin rashes from sunscreen:*

- Benzophenone
- Methoxycinnamate
- Padimate
- Para-aminobenzoic acid (PABA)

## Your Makeup

In choosing makeup products, avoid any that contain the ingredients listed above. You should also stay away from shimmery shadows, since these products may contain pieces of shell that will irritate dry, sensitive skin. D and C red dyes in blush and color makeup can lead to acne, so if you tend to break out over the cheek area, make sure your cosmetics do not contain these dyes. There are many types of D and C red dyes but the xanthenes, mono-azoanilines, fluorans, and indigoids are the most problematic.

### RECOMMENDED FOUNDATIONS

- $ CoverGirl's CG Smoothers Tinted Moisturizer SPF 15
- $ Mary Kay Full Coverage Foundation
- $$ Kevyn Aucoin Dew Drop Foundation
- $$ Laura Geller Balance-n-Brighten Compact
- $$ Trish McEvoy Protective Shield Tinted Moisturizer
- $$$ M·A·C Studio Fix Fluid Foundation SPF 15

**Baumann's Choice:** CoverGirl's CG Smoothers Tinted Moisturizer SPF 15—I first heard about it from another DSNT at www.skintype solutions.com.

### RECOMMENDED CREAM EYESHADOWS

- $ Almay Bright Eyes
- $ Revlon Illuminance Creme Shadow
- $$ Bliss Lidthicks
- $$ Bobbi Brown Cream Shadow Stick
- $$ Clinique Touch Tint for Eyes Cream Formula

**Baumann's Choice:** Bliss Lidthicks with antioxidants

## RECOMMENDED BLUSHES

$  CoverGirl Tru Blend Minerals Blush
$  Mary Kay Mineral Cheek Color
$$  Biotherm BLUSH!
$$  Bobbi Brown Cream Blush Stick
$$  Jane Iredale Blush (powder blush with soothing minerals)
$$  M·A·C Cosmetics Beauty Powder Blush

**Baumann's Choice:** They are all good.


## PROCEDURES FOR YOUR SKIN TYPE

Your type does not need any skin care procedures. However, for some problems, you may wish to consult a dermatologist. For example, if your skin reacts to multiple skin care products, your dermatologist can patch test you to find out whether you are indeed allergic and, if so, precisely what you are allergic to. Patch testing involves taping small samples of several types of allergens on your back. You return to the doctor twenty-four hours later to see if any of the areas have developed redness, which indicates an allergic reaction. Sometimes several tests, using different allergens, are needed before you can find out what is causing your allergy.


## ONGOING CARE FOR YOUR SKIN

Avoid harsh chemicals, environmental extremes, and anything that could undermine your skin barrier. Moisturize continually and spray water before moisturizer use. Make sure to incorporate essential fats into your diet, because repairing and maintaining a healthy skin barrier is your first priority.

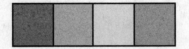

## PART FIVE

# Skin Care for Dry, Resistant Skin

# CHAPTER SIXTEEN

# Dry, Resistant, Pigmented, and Wrinkled: DRPW

## BAUMANN SKIN TYPE NUMBER 15

■

*"I have found many products that feel good on my skin and they all seem alike to me. However, I am not convinced that they are the best products to improve my wrinkles and uneven complexion."*

### ABOUT YOUR SKIN

I love DRPWs because there is so much that I can do to help your skin. And my DRPW patients are grateful for what cosmetic dermatology can offer. Younger DRPWs rarely consult a dermatologist, so I usually see this type once the signs of aging have appeared.

With DRPW skin, wrinkles are the chief complaint. Your skin may feel tight, rough to the touch, and even sore, especially in drying environmental conditions, such as on an airplane or in a low-humidity environment like Colorado. In the winter, when indoor heating is used, your skin gets even more dehydrated, making the wrinkles look worse. Your skin may catch on wool and other rough clothing. You may also notice wrinkles on your hands.

Older DRPWs come into my office, desperate to address the skin wrinkling, and they feel a lot of regret. Although genes certainly play a role in everyone's skin condition, for DRPWs, decades of neglect, or even mistreatment, of their skin is most frequently the source of their skin problems. Many say that if they knew then what they know now, they would have done it differently. That's why I want to alert DRPWs young and old to take steps now to protect your skin and prevent wrinkles.

You are the type that goes for a day of fun on the beach without sun protection, who sails or skis without moisturizing against the harsh winds or blasting cold. You head out without a hat, figuring your easy-to-tan skin can handle anything. Many of you prefer to be active, rather than take the time to mess around with beauty stuff.

On a daily basis, you may rarely wear sunscreen, use any old moisturizer, and wash with drying soaps. You wouldn't wear foundation to save your life. You shrug off antiaging treatments. You can't be bothered. Most of you fail to protect your skin, and your dry skin can't take the abuse. As early as your early thirties, and increasingly as you get older, the signs of aging appear and accelerate. At first, you try to ignore the wrinkles, pretending they don't matter. Soon you can't ignore them, but you still don't like to admit that your obvious skin problems *are* problems. Once you admit that they upset you, you believe that it's too late. "I just have to grin and bear it," one DRPW patient shrugged and told me. Overnight, the carefree go-for-it girl or guy becomes the resigned, prematurely aging woman or man. Skin problems sneak up on you, and once they manifest, many of you just give up.

But you *can* do something about it, whatever your age. If you are an older DRPW, don't give up, I can help even you. And if you are a younger DRPW, take heed and act now to prevent the worst downsides of your type.

## THE HARSH REALITY OF DRPW SKIN

During their teens and twenties, DRPWs have great skin. Unlike oily types, you experience no acne. Unlike sensitive types, you have no problems using skin care products and ingredients. As far as pigment goes, there are two types of DRPWs: the fair-skinned and freckled who don't tan well and the people who can easily achieve the Hawaiian tropic tan. If you're in the latter group, you may often fail to use sunscreen regularly. Fair-skinned DRPWs may have frequently burned trying to achieve that unobtainable tan, attaining instead only freckles and peeling skin.

For women, the first problems crop up in their twenties or thirties, the age when many get pregnant or take birth control pills. Dark spots and dark under-eye circles may result. In your early thirties, you may develop lines around your eyes and between your eyebrows. DRPWs often develop both lines underneath the eyes just below the lower lids and under-eye dark circles. Your skin's dryness makes the wrinkles even more noticeable. Moisturizers are absorbed quickly, providing only minimal hydration. With age (and menopause), skin dryness and wrinkles worsen.

Though some DRPWs abuse their skin through sunning, smoking, and poor dietary habits, you (along with many other DRPWs) may not have abused your skin, but are trying to overcome a genetic tendency to wrinkle. Your best chance is to do everything possible to tip the scales in your favor. A little sun here, a cigarette occasionally at a party, an occasional indulgence in junk food may not be the worst thing in the world for many types, but you cannot afford it. In a high-risk group, you must do everything right to limit visible aging. Follow my preventive strategies whenever possible.

DRPWs have some of the most dreaded skin issues. Wrinkles, sags, premature aging, dryness, dark spots, flaking, and peeling skin result from years of disregard. By the time you reach your late forties and fifties, your skin's wrinkling and dryness may make you feel like giving up on your skin in frustration.

At any age, knowing how to protect, hydrate, and moisturize your skin is key. For those of you who are starting early in the game—congratulations. If you use sunscreen, include antioxidants (obtained via foods, supplements, and topical products), and learn how to protect and moisturize, chances are excellent that you can moderate your skin's tendency to wrinkle.

For older DRPWs, there's still much that can be done. After all, chances are you have another twenty to forty years left to live with your skin, so it's never too late to begin.

## SUNTANNING

Many people with this Skin Type (or its close cousin, the DRPT Skin Type) may have a medium skin tone and tan well.

Sun exposure worsens dry skin, and you are one of the types most vulnerable to sun-induced aging. The UV rays inhibit skin enzymes that produce key components in your skin, and thus damage your skin's ability to hold on to water. That's why sunburned skin flakes and peels off, and this damage can lead to ongoing dryness and flaking. Sun exposure also decreases the skin's hyaluronic acid (HA) content. HA is a chain of sugars that draws water into the skin and plumps it up, giving it volume. Sun-damaged skin tends to have less volume to it due in part to a loss of HA. Sun stimulates the cells to produce melanin, the skin pigment that makes dark spots and freckles.

Some dry, resistant types can feel the sun's drying effect and naturally avoid sun exposure. However, they are more likely to test as tight types, especially if they've avoided the sun their entire lives. I, too, have dry skin, and always protect my skin, a habit I learned from my mom, who is a DSNT like me. My mother was a smoker for many years and could have easily wound up a non-pigmented, wrinkled type rather than a non-pigmented, tight type except that she didn't care for the sun because her non-pigmented skin burned. To me, she's a clear example of how even a single lifestyle factor can change your type.

Sunscreen use is essential to protect against wrinkles and dark spots. Apply it to your face and to the backs of your hands. Purchase a sunscreen that blocks both UVB (which give you a tan) *and* UVA rays (more insidious because they penetrate more deeply into the skin, initiating a collagen breakdown cascade that will ultimately produce wrinkles).

## YOUR MELANOMA RISK

Although you are less likely to get non-melanoma skin cancer than non-pigmented types, light-skinned DRPWs are at greatest risk for developing melanoma skin cancers, which are curable when detected early. Make sure to get annual dermatology checkups, especially if you have frequently sunburned. Light treatments offered by a dermatologist can easily remove any worrisome spots that could develop into non-melanoma skin cancers but it's still important to know your risk factors and get an annual skin cancer exam to look for melanoma lesions.

If you're a DRPW with several of the following factors, you are at higher risk of developing melanoma:

- Light skin
- Sunburn easily
- History of one or more severe sunburns
- Many freckles
- Family members with history of melanoma

While all light-skinned DRPWs should pay heed, any of the above factors will increase your risk. In addition, if you have red hair, your risk *further* increases. Here's why: The MC1R gene is involved in red hair, freckle, and melanoma formation, research reveals. Bottom line? Freckles are not just a cosmetic concern. They may be an early warning sign of the potential for future skin cancers. A landmark study published in the *Journal of the American Medical Association* showed that children who used sunscreen developed fewer freckles. While some consider freckles "cute," their presence may indicate an increased melanoma risk. Any mole that grows suddenly; changes in size, shape, or color; or bleeds should be seen by a dermatologist immediately. In addition to checking your skin frequently, wear protective clothing and sunscreen when possible. Please consult "The A, B, C, and D of Melanoma" in Chapter Nine for a complete description of what to look out for.

The lip area is most prone to skin cancer because the lips do not secrete sebum, which contains a high concentration of vitamin E, an antioxidant that protects against aging and cancer. That's why some formulations of Chap Stick and lip balm contain vitamin E as a protectant. Health food stores also sell vitamin E oil, which, though too oily for most skin areas, can be used on the lips.

## A CLOSE-UP LOOK AT YOUR SKIN

With DRPW skin you may experience any of the following:

- Dry flaking skin
- Itching
- Thin skin with easy tearing of the skin if you are over fifty
- Easy bruising of the skin
- Dark spots on face, chest, arms, and hands
- Wrinkles beginning around the eyes
- Wrinkles on the forehead and between the eyebrows
- Wrinkled hands
- Higher risk of melanoma skin cancer

Aged skin is more likely to be dry. In addition, dry skin is more susceptible to skin aging for several reasons. First, skin enzymes that repair skin damage function less efficiently in skin with a lower water content. Second, dry types produce less sebum, an oily substance that contains large amounts of vitamin E, a skin protective antioxidant that combats aging and skin cancer. Third, the cell cycle (which produces new skin cells) slows down, causing dead skin cells to pile up in little hills and valleys. Though not visible to the naked eye, these make the skin appear rough. Finally, when estrogen levels decline with perimenopause and menopause, the skin becomes drier.

## TREATING WRINKLES

Yours is an underserved Skin Type. You experiment with various skin care products, but nothing seems to make a difference. In general, over-the-counter products are not strong enough because companies don't offer products with higher concentrations of effective ingredients, because they can't regulate who purchases their products. They compromise and offer lower-strength products that anyone can safely use without side effects.

In any case, until more powerful over-the-counter products are offered, you can use stronger prescription products. Your skin can deal with them. However, you must commit to consistent sunscreen use to protect your skin, because retinoid prescription medication may allow increased penetration of the sun's harmful sun rays. Despite this, in my opinion, it's the most valuable product for DRPW skin because it prevents wrinkles and dark spots, and even helps to eliminate existing dark spots and some fine wrinkles. Buy the cheapest cleansers and sunscreens, because your resistant skin does not require babying. Instead, save your money for prescription medications like retinoids that really do the job.

## Retinols and DRPWs

To prevent or minimize the wrinkles to which this type is prone, many DRPWs use retinol in over-the-counter cosmetics or Retin-A in prescription formulations. They both work the same way, by increasing cell renewal and preventing the breakdown in collagen, which is a key contributor to skin aging.

Which is right for you? Here are the pros and cons.

On the one hand, most nonprescription retinol-containing products are not sufficiently concentrated to completely address all your spots or wrinkles. Retinol is very unstable. If in the manufacturing or packaging process it's exposed to air or light, it will be rendered ineffective. The packaging itself must keep the product protected from light, which is why aluminum tubes are frequently used. A retinol product offered in a clear jar or bottle is inactive. That's why my product recommendations list creams that I know are produced and packaged in the right way. If you are starting young and have not yet begun to see wrinkles (or if your wrinkles are just beginning to show), they may help. However, you may find that they are not strong enough and that you need to graduate to prescription-strength products, especially if you have many visible wrinkles already.

Many DRPWs have trouble with prescription-strength products because they cannot tolerate the dryness and flaking that result from the full-strength retinoids.

Still, for you I maintain that a retinoid prescription product will give the best value especially if you introduce its use slowly and dilute it with a moisturizer, if needed, to prevent irritation. Most antiaging creams will either not contain sufficient quantities of active ingredients or, if they are potent enough, they will most likely be expensive (over $200) because of the high cost of these ingredients. A $90 prescription of Avage cream would do more for you. Add the onetime cost of a doctor visit (assuming your insurance does not cover it) of $190 and you still come out cheaper on the second tube of Avage. The prescriptions usually last for one year.

## Wrinkle Prevention

In addition to using retinoids, antioxidants are another vital ingredient in your antiwrinkle campaign because they block the harmful effects of free radicals. Free radicals are oxygen molecules that have an odd number of electrons. They like to have an even number, so they "steal" electrons from vital skin components such as DNA and cell membrane lipids. Losing the electron damages the DNA or cell membrane lipids, leading to skin cancers and aging.

Although antioxidant green tea has been proven beneficial to the skin, many products contain such low amounts that they are near to worthless. Green tea turns brown when used in large amounts; as a result, companies often put in only small quantities. The products I'll recommend that are brown contain higher quantities of green tea. Don't let the brown color worry you. Think about the benefit to your skin.

L-ascorbic acid, or vitamin C, is another important antioxidant in the skin. Studies have shown that it both prevents the breakdown of collagen *and* increases collagen production. However, vitamin C comes in many forms, and not all of them are helpful. Vitamin C esters attached to a fatty acid are poorly absorbed into the skin when applied topically, so products that contain this form of vitamin C are not that effective, while certain other forms of vitamin C, such as L-ascorbic acid, penetrate the skin more readily. That's why I'll be recommending vitamin C–containing products that really work.

To combat dryness, topical estrogen creams and soy-containing products are an option for female postmenopausal DRPWs who do not opt for hormone replacement therapy. Fortunately, there are also many new technologies that can help treat the problems common to this type.

If wrinkles have already appeared, you need it all. And if you feel distressed at having to go to such lengths to retain a youthful appearance, consider this: Thankfully, you are not a sensitive type, which means that your resistant skin can handle the strong stuff.

**Dr. Baumann's Bottom Line:** Spend the money to see a dermatologist. It will save you money in the long run. If you go to a spa, forget the facial treatments and get a massage. They can't do anything strong enough to help you—but I can.

## EVERYDAY CARE FOR YOUR SKIN TYPE

The goal of your skin care routine is to address wrinkles, dark spots, and dryness with products that deliver lightening, moisturizing, and antiwrinkle ingredients.

Your daily regimen is based on protecting, hydrating, and moisturizing your dry skin. But since your skin is resistant, you need strong ingredients to treat your wrinkles and dark spots.

I've provided two regimens for you, the first for when you have no dark spots and the second for when you do. I know that many of you will first want to try the dark-spots regimen.

If you can afford it, go straight to your dermatologist, who can prescribe the strong products that may really work for you.

### DAILY SKIN CARE

---

### REGIMEN FOR WHEN YOU HAVE NO SPOTS:

| AM | PM |
|---|---|
| Step 1: Wash with cleanser | Step 1: Wash with cleanser |
| Step 2: Apply eye cream | Step 2: Use an exfoliator |
| Step 3: Apply antiaging serum to face, neck, and chest | Step 3: Apply eye cream |
| | Step 4: Apply a retinol-containing moisturizer |

Step 4: Apply moisturizer with sunscreen to face, neck, and chest

Step 5: Apply a moisturizer

Step 5: Apply foundation (optional)

In the morning, wash with cleanser, then apply eye cream. Next, apply an antiaging serum to your face, neck, and chest. Apply moisturizer and/or sunscreen, and then finish with foundation if you wish to use one. Assure you attain an SPF of 15 or more from the products you use.

In the evening, wash with cleanser. Then, once a week, use microdermabrasion or an exfoliating scrub as your second step. Look for options and instructions under "Exfoliation." Next, apply eye cream, and then a night cream containing retinol. Finish with a moisturizer.

## REGIMEN TO GET RID OF DARK SPOTS:

### AM

Step 1: Wash with cleanser

Step 2: Apply eye cream

Step 3: Apply lightening serum or gel to dark spots

Step 4: Apply moisturizer with sunscreen

Step 5: Apply foundation (optional)

### PM

Step 1: Wash with cleanser

Step 2: Use an exfoliator

Step 3: Apply eye cream

Step 4: Apply lightening serum or gel to dark spots

Step 5: Apply moisturizer containing retinol

Step 6: Apply night cream

In the morning, wash with cleanser, then apply eye cream. Next, apply lightening serum or gel to your dark spots. Then apply moisturizer with SPF to your face, neck, and chest. Finally, apply foundation if you choose. Make sure your product selection provides a minimum SPF of 15.

In the evening, wash with cleanser. Then, use an exfoliating scrub or microdermabrasion kit one to four times a week (see instructions under "Exfoliation" in this chapter). Apply eye cream, then apply a lightening serum or gel to your dark spots. Next, apply a moisturizer containing retinol. Finish with a night cream.

There's one more option you can try to get rid of resistant dark spots before seeing your dermatologist. It's the Alpha Beta Daily Face Peel by Dr. Dennis Gross, which you can find at www.mdskincare.com. Use it once daily as the second step of the regimen. (In that case, Step 2 would become Step 3, and so on.) If after one week, you experience no redness or irritation, you can use it twice a day.

## Cleansers

DRPWs benefit from cleansers containing ingredients like glycolic acid that hydrate, exfoliate, and moisturize the skin, as well as antioxidants that help prevent wrinkles. However, recent research suggests that alpha hydroxy acids (AHA) may make the skin more sensitive to sunlight. So if you are out in the sun a lot and tend to be lax about sunscreen use, you may not want to use a glycolic acid cleanser. In that case, my next choice is Vichy Rich Detoxifying Cleansing Milk.

### RECOMMENDED CLEANSING PRODUCTS

- $ Gly Derm Gentle Cleanser (has glycolic acid 2%)
- $$ Aveeno Skin Brightening Daily Scrub
- $$ Glycolix Elite 10% Moisturizing Cleanser (Has 10% glycolic acid)
- $$ Vivite Exfoliating Facial Cleanser
- $$ M.D. Forté Facial Cleanser (Start with I and slowly move up to II and then III)
- $$ Nia24 Physical Cleansing Scrub
- $$ Vichy Rich Detoxifying Cleansing Milk
- $$$ Derma 24 C Daily Vitamins Healthy Skin Facial Cleanser

**Baumann's Choice:** Vivite Exfoliating Facial Cleanser because it has glycolic acid, as well as a light polishing ingredient. Twice a day may be too often because it contains some salicylic acid that may dry skin.

## Serums and Emulsions

These products should contain antioxidants or skin lighteners to treat dark spots. I never thought I would find a vitamin C product that I could recommend until recent advances resulted in the development of La Roche-Posay Active C and others that are perfect for your Skin Type. The vitamin C reduces pigment and increases collagen production to improve and treat wrinkles.

### RECOMMENDED SERUMS AND EMULSIONS

- $ RoC Multi-Correxion Skin Renewing Serum
- $ Olay Pro X Skin Tightening Serum
- $$ La Roche-Posay Active C for Dry Skin
- $$ iS Clinical Super Serum Advance+
- $$ Replenix Power of 3 Cream
- $$ Vichy Reti-C
- $$$ Boske Dermaceuticals Alchemist C Serum
- $$$ SkinCeuticals C E Ferulic
- $$$ Combray Serum by Solenne

**Baumann's Choice:** Combray Serum by Solenne

## Moisturizers

Your moisturizer and eye cream should contain hydrating, lightening, and antioxidant ingredients. In addition, your daytime moisturizer should contain sunscreen.

### RECOMMENDED DAYTIME MOISTURIZERS

- $ Neutrogena Healthy Skin Visible Even Daily SPF15 Moisturizer
- $ Aveeno Positively Radiant Daily Moisturizing Lotion SPF 15 or 30
- $$ Elizabeth Arden Intervene Moisture Cream SPF 15
- $$ Philosophy When Hope Is Not Enough Cream SPF 20
- $$ Pevonia Glycocides Cream
- $$ Vichy Aqualia Thermal Lotion SPF 30 Fortifying & Soothing 24Hr Hydrating Moisturizer

$$$ Bobbi Brown Extra SPF 25 Moisturizing Balm
$$$ La Prairie Cellular Moisturizer Face

**Baumann's Choice:** Elizabeth Arden Intervene Moisture Cream SPF 15

### RECOMMENDED NIGHT CREAMS

$ Aveeno Ageless Vitality Restorative Night Treatment
$ Eucerin Sensitive Facial Skin $Q_{10}$ Anti-Wrinkle Sensitive Skin Cream
$ Skin Effects Cell 2 Cell Intense Illuminated Cream
$$ Reviva Labs EFAs Cream
$$ Korres Quercetin and Oak Antiageing and Antiwrinkle Night Cream
$$ Kiehl's Lycopene Facial Moisturizing Cream
$$ L'Occitane en Provence Brightening Immortelle Moisture Cream
$$ Vivite Night Renewal Facial Cream
$$ AtoPalm MLE cream (In the jar, not the tube)
$$ Nia24 Intensive Recovery Complex
$$ Crème de la Mer

**Baumann's Choice:** Vivite Night Renewal Facial Cream if you are not going to use a retinol-containing product

### RECOMMENDED EVENING MOISTURIZERS CONTAINING RETINOL

$ Neutrogena Ageless Intensives Deep Wrinkle Moisture
$$ RoC Retinol Correxion Deep Wrinkle Night Cream
$$ Afirm 3x
$$ La Roche-Posay BioMedic Retinol 60
$$ SkinCeuticals Retinol 1.0
$$ Topix Replenix Retinol Smoothing Serum 5X

**Baumann's Choice:** I like all these products.

### RECOMMENDED EYE CREAMS

$ Neutrogena Clinical Eye Lift Contouring Treatment
$ Aveeno Ageless Vitality Revitalizing Eye Treatment
$ Skineffects by Dr. Jeffrey Dover Intensive Eye Treatment with Vitamin C

$$ Kinerase Ultra Rich Eye Repair
$$ Laura Mercier Eyedration Firming Eye Cream
$$ La Roche-Posay Active-C Eyes
$$ Origins Eye Doctor
$$ Relastin Eye Silk
$$$ M.D. Forté Skin Rejuvenation Eye Cream

**Baumann's Choice:** Kinerase Ultra Rich Eye Repair

## Exfoliation

Use a scrub or microdermabrasion kit once, then wait a week to see how you tolerate it. If your skin does not become red or feel tender, use the kit two times the next week. After two weeks you can move to three times a week. Very resistant skin may even be able to tolerate microdermabrasion creams or scrubs four times a week, but in most cases this will be too irritating.

As an alternative to home care, you can go to a spa for an exfoliation treatment. Be sure your spa services professional uses an exfoliator with antioxidant ingredients.

### RECOMMENDED MICRODERMABRASION OR EXFOLIATION KITS

$ Skin Effects Cell 2 Cell Anti-Aging Exfoliating Cleansing Scrub
$ Origins Modern Friction
$ Vivite Exfoliating Cleanser
$$ Ahava Gentle Mud Exfoliator
$$ Clinique 7 Day Scrub Cream
$$ Neova Microdermabrasion Scrub
$$ Philosophy the Microdelivery Micro-Massage Exfoliating Wash
$$$ Dr. Brandt Microdermabrasion in a Jar

**Baumann's Choice:** Vivite Exfoliating Cleanser

## SHOPPING FOR PRODUCTS

With resistant skin, should you wish to, you can widen your selection from the products I specifically recommend. Look for products that contain the recommended ingredients and where those you should avoid are minimal. If you find a favorite product that contains these ingredients but is not on my list of recommendations, please go to www.skintypesolutions.com and share it with me.

## RECOMMENDED SKIN CARE INGREDIENTS

### To prevent wrinkles:

- Basil
- Caffeine
- *Camilla sinensis* (green tea, white tea)
- Coenzyme $Q_{10}$ (ubiquinone)
- Copper peptide
- Curcumin (tetrahydracurcumin or turmeric)
- Ferulic acid
- Feverfew
- Ginger
- Ginseng
- Grape seed extract
- Idebenone
- Lutein
- Lycopene
- *Punica granatum* (pomegranate)
- Pycnogenol (a pine bark extract)
- Rosemary
- Silymarin
- Vitamin C
- Vitamin E
- Yucca

### To improve the appearance of wrinkles:

- Alpha hydroxy acids (glycolic acid, lactic acid)
- DMAE
- Retinol
- Vitamin C (ascorbic acid)

### To moisturize:

- Aloe vera
- Borage seed oil
- Ceramide
- Cholesterol
- Cocoa butter
- Colloidal oatmeal
- Dexpanthenol (pro-vitamin $B_5$)
- Dimethicone
- Evening primrose oil
- Glycerin
- Glycolic acid
- Jojoba oil
- Lactic acid
- Linoleic acid
- Niacinamide
- Olive oil
- Safflower oil
- Shea butter

*To prevent dark spots:*

- *Cocos nucifera* (coconut extract)
- Cucumber
- Niacinamide

- Pycnogenol (a pine bark extract)
- *Saxifraga sarmentosa* extract (strawberry begonia)

*To improve dark spots:*

- Arbutin
- Cucumber extract
- *Glycyrrhiza glabra* (licorice extract)
- Hydroquinone
- Kojic acid

- Magnesium ascorbyl phosphate
- Mulberry extract
- Tyrostat
- Vitamin C (ascorbic acid)

**SKIN CARE INGREDIENTS TO AVOID:**

- Alcohol

- Detergents that foam vigorously

Alcohol, often used as an ingredient in skin care, can increase dryness. However, not every kind of alcohol is a problem. A glycol is a beneficial alcohol that increases the penetration of other ingredients. But alcohol that has a low molecular weight, such as ethanol, denatured alcohol, ethyl alcohol, methanol, benzyl alcohol, isopropyl alcohol, and SD alcohol, should be avoided.

## Sun Protection for Your Skin

Whenever you're in the sun for longer than fifteen minutes, you need extra protection, over and above your everyday SPF. So at those times of longer exposure, layer on a sunscreen that is SPF 45 or more. For DRPWs, I suggest cream or lotion sunscreens. If your skin is very dry, use cream; if it's only slightly dry, use lotion. Fortunately for you, there are no sunscreen ingredients you need to avoid.

Studies show most people apply only a quarter of the amount of sunscreen that they need. If a high price will make you unwilling to apply a large amount, avoid expensive sunscreens: You need to use about a quarter-size dollop on each exposed area, your face, neck, and chest. Make sure the combined SPF of all products you use during the day, such as moisturizer, sunscreen, and foundation, will provide an SPF of at least 15.

### RECOMMENDED SUN PROTECTION PRODUCTS

$ Eucerin Sensitive Facial Skin Extra Protective Moisture Lotion with SPF 30

$ Blue Lizard Australian Suncream Regular SPF 30+

$ Neutrogena Ultra Sheer Dry-Touch Sunblock SPF 55, 70, & 85

$$ SkinCeuticals Ultimate UV Defense SPF 30

$$$ Darphin Vital Protection Age-Defying Protective Lotion SPF 15

$$$ Nia24 Sun Damage Prevention 100% Mineral Sunscreen

$$$ Yonka Ultra Protection SPF 25

**Baumann's Choice:** Blue Lizard Australian Suncream Regular SPF 30+ or choose the baby version if you prefer a chemical-free sunscreen.

## Your Makeup

Wait a few minutes after applying sunscreen to apply foundation or other cosmetic products. This gives your sunscreen time to soak in. If you have very dry skin, look for cream eyeshadows and blushes. A nice cream eye shadow for your type is Laura Mercier Metallic Creme Eye Colour. Avoid powders, which will make your skin look drier.

### RECOMMENDED FOUNDATIONS

$ Boots No7 True Identity Foundation

$ Revlon ColorStay Makeup with SoftFlex SPF 15 for Normal/Dry Skin

$$ Awake Skin Renovation Foundation

$$ Chantecaille Real Skin Foundation SPF 30 for Dry Skin

$$ Laura Mercier Tinted Moisturizer

$$ Makeup Forever Professional HD Invisible Cover Foundation

$$$ La Prairie Cellular Treatment Foundation

**Baumann's Choice:** Revlon ColorStay Makeup with SoftFlex SPF 15 for Normal/Dry Skin

## PROCEDURES FOR YOUR SKIN TYPE

In my experience, most DRPWs with medium to dark skin tones can best treat their dark spots with prescription topical products and chemical peels. Lasers and light treatments cannot be used on dark skin, since these procedures can lead to inflammation and worsening, or development, of dark spots. People with resistant, pigmented skin are at an advantage over SP types, because they can use stronger ingredients without fear of sensitivity, and these stronger ingredients may work faster. Still, you should expect to wait about four to six weeks to see improvement.

DRPWs with light skin have the added option of skin procedures such as laser and light therapy to lighten the dark spots without causing inflammation that leads to more dark spots.

For wrinkle treatment, both lighter- and darker-skinned DRPWs can benefit from botulinum toxin injections and dermal fillers.

Lighter-skinned DRPWs also have the option of dermabrasion, a resurfacing treatment for lines around the mouth. This method requires an experienced physician. For more details on the procedure and finding physicians who can perform it, see "Dermabrasion" in the procedures section of Chapter Ten. Thermage, a new technology used to treat droopy skin on the face and neck, is also appropriate for your skin type.

## ONGOING CARE FOR YOUR SKIN

Protect—and moisturize without delay—every day. Pay attention to prevention now and eat an antioxidant-rich diet. Although aging well is one of your chief challenges, many new technologies can help address your problems. See a dermatologist. You'll never regret it.

# CHAPTER SEVENTEEN

# Dry, Resistant, Pigmented, and Tight: DRPT

## BAUMANN SKIN TYPE NUMBER 13

∎

*"My darker skin is dry, but luckily I rarely suffer from acne or redness. My goal is a smoother, even toned, and radiant complexion. I want good products but I do not want to waste money on unnecessary products."*

## ABOUT YOUR SKIN

If your questionnaire results revealed you as a DRPT, you share this Skin Type with many beautiful women from every place on this planet. Italian icons, like Sophia Loren; Asian stunners, like Lucy Liu; gorgeous women of color, like Halle Berry; and striking Spanish beauties like Penelope Cruz all have that golden-toned DRPT skin. Although not every DRPT will be blessed with their gorgeous, rich skin color, nearly every ethnic group can have this Skin Type. Though less common among Caucasians of northern European background, this Skin Type can occur among all groups, making it one of the most universal.

Your smooth, ageless skin is the envy of other types who struggle with wrinkles. You're rarely troubled with oiliness and outbreaks, and pass through your teens and twenties unconcerned. Though your skin may grow slightly drier as you age, this can be easily addressed since your resistant skin can readily handle products that other types must avoid.

Although light- and medium-toned DRPTs tan quite well due to their moderate to high pigment levels, tanning can cause wrinkles, dark spots, and melasma, and is best avoided. Most of you have gotten the message to shun excess sun exposure. Along with good genes and a healthy diet, that's why you enjoy the blessings of tight skin.

Constant moisture will help preserve your skin's youthful qualities. Be vigilant to protect your skin from the elements and use non-drying products.

Tight skin results from a combination of lifestyle factors and genes, and for the majority of DRPTs, good genes play a major part. In medium- to dark-skin-toned people, resistant, highly pigmented skin tends to wrinkle less. It has more resilience and lifelong elasticity than lighter-toned skin. For lighter-skinned people who scored as DRPTs, lifestyle factors play a bigger role in maintaining your skin tightness. Using moisturizers, avoiding the sun, eating antioxidant-filled fruits and vegetables, never smoking, protecting your skin from drying environments like chlorine pools, hot rooms, cold winds, drying climes, steam baths, and even facials are key to maintaining your dry, tight skin.

## PIGMENTATION AND YOUR SKIN

While this Skin Type is common among people with medium and darker skin tones, some DRPTs do have light skin with many skin areas showing signs of pigmentation, such as dark spots, freckles, melasma, or sun spots. If you're an Irish redhead with a tendency to freckle, don't retake the test; this can be your type as well. What you all have in common is the tendency to pigment. Redheads may have trouble getting a tan but they easily freckle. Darker-skinned DRPTs tan easily but are more susceptible to dark spots.

Many people consider freckles attractive, but there are a wide variety of other ways that higher pigment levels show up, and they aren't so pretty. Pigmentation and skin dryness may interact to give you rough, dark, dry patches over the knees and elbows. No amount of scrubbing with soap and water will remove these "dirty"-looking areas.

Dark raised bumps may appear on the backs of your arms and on the sides of your thighs. Called keratosis pilaris, these unsightly bumps, which are about the size of a pinpoint, are produced by friction and skin dryness. Your parents or siblings likely have them too, as they can run in families.

You're also susceptible to developing dark spots on your face, especially when you are pregnant, on oral contraceptives, or hormone replacement therapy, as higher estrogen levels make melanocytes produce more melanin (skin pigment). For both men and women, sun exposure can instigate freckles or sun spots anywhere on the body. When these appear on the hands, they're called liver spots.

Dark patches can result from skin traumas, such as cuts, ingrown hairs, or pimples, as well as heat exposure. In low humidity and cold, your dry skin gets even drier, especially on your arms and legs. When exceptionally dry, your skin may itch. Dry skin worsens with age, which is why preserving skin moisture and hydration is crucial.

Dark spots, patches, and melasma all result from high pigment levels. Dryness, rough fabrics, or any form of heat, irritation, or inflammation will stimulate their formation.

Light-skinned DRPTs can benefit from dermatological procedures to treat dark spots, while medium-, dark-, and Asian-skinned people should follow my product recommendations for dark skin.

Finally, thick, velvety-looking dark patches that appear *under* the arms could be a skin disorder called acanthosis nigricans, which is most common in overweight people. The skin-lightening ingredients I'll offer will not treat this condition. Instead, see your physician.

## A CLOSE-UP LOOK AT YOUR SKIN

With DRPT skin you may experience:

- Dry skin
- Rough patches over the knees and elbows that appear darker than the rest of your skin
- Freckles or sun spots
- Dark patches on cheeks (such as melasma, or mask of pregnancy)
- Dark eye circles, giving you a raccoon-like appearance
- Dark areas in site of previous injury or inflammation, such as a cut, pimple, or scrape
- Itching skin
- Flaking skin
- Chemical peels or other treatments worsen dark spots

Under-eye circles are quite common, caused by decreased (or congested) blood flow, which is thought to result in the deposit under the eyes of a substance called hemisiderin, which also appears in bruised skin, causing the purplish color. Beneficial eye creams will include vitamin K or arnica, which address dark circles by speeding up the rate at which the purplish cast clears.

Over time, some DRPT skin issues worsen while others improve. Women experience a lessening of melasma when estrogen levels drop due to midlife changes. On the other hand, freckles and sun spots increase with age, as does drying, which often worsens after menopause.

## DRPTs AROUND THE WORLD

The DRPT Skin Type is quite common in Latin America. In Venezuela, sun protection is deeply ingrained. Children as young as five learn to use sunscreen regularly. Venezuelan women prize clear complexions, wrinkle-free, and spot-free skin. The Venezuelans admire and respect beauty—so much so that the woman crowned as Miss Venezuela can sometimes wind up being elected to a high political office after her reign is over.

Latina DRPTs prefer not to wash with soap and water because they know it dries their skin. They use oil-based cleansers, which they wipe off with a cloth, creating a mild exfoliation, which DRPT skin can handle.

The majority of Asians are pigmented types, and fall into the DRPT and DSPT categories. Many Asians complain of oily skin, but when I measure their surface skin oil, they most often are dry types, revealing that it's hard for people to accurately assess their own skin. Asians are less concerned with wrinkling than with dark-spot treatment, a major emphasis in product offerings for the Asian market. Hydroquinone, commonly used in American skin lighteners, is illegal in Europe and Asia, because in certain rare instances, prolonged exposure has resulted in damage to the cornea. For some reason, Asians are also more vulnerable to developing pigmentation problems after long-term use. That's why in Asia and elsewhere, other ingredients, such as kojic acid, are used to lighten skin. To offset any potential problem arising from long-term use, I advise using hydroquinone-containing products in four-month cycles, alternating with kojic acid, azelaic acid, and other bleaching agents.

## BLACK DRPTs

DRPTs with dark-toned skin are prone to develop "ashiness," which is a gray appearance caused by flaking skin lighter in color than the dark-toned skin showing through underneath. Common to many dry-skinned people of color, this skin problem can be easily treated with a moisturizer, though there are many products marketed directly for it as well.

Dark spots in response to injury trouble many dark-skinned DRPTs because skin pigmentation developed at the site of injury may last much longer than the injury itself. Black patients frequently fear that these dark spots are permanent scars, but they are neither permanent nor scars. However, you may have a harder time getting rid of the dark spots than light-skin-toned DRPTs. Light treatments (commonly used to treat them) are not useful for you because the light can affect your overall skin color pigment as well as the spot you want to remove. Instead, you'll have to rely on the products I recommend. When my black and Asian patients are upset because they cannot avail themselves of these procedures, I remind them that their cancer risk is much lower than it is for light-skin-toned DRPTs. It's a trade-off.

With dark-toned DRPT skin you may experience any of the following:

- Dry skin
- Rough patches over the knees and elbows that appear darker than the rest of your skin
- Dark patches on the cheek (such as melasma, or mask of pregnancy)
- Dark areas in site of previous injury or inflammation, such as a cut, pimple, or scrape
- Itching skin
- Ashiness
- Flaking skin
- Chemical peels or other treatments worsen dark spots

If your skin measures very dry on the questionnaire, you may develop dryness, dandruff, and peeling all over your face and head as well. For people of color, often dryness is worsened by harsh hair products. Unlike those with sensitive skin, resistant types do not always develop reactions (such as rashes or itching) to these ingredients, but you still can find them very drying. While hair care products are outside the scope of this book, if you notice that you're developing extreme dryness and dandruff, I would suggest that you seek out milder products, avoiding shampoos and conditioners that contain detergents, and steer clear of hair straighteners, hair growth products, hair dyes, and professional treatments with harsh chemicals. You might also consider spacing out your hair appointments to minimize exposure.

## YOUR MELANOMA RISK

Light-skinned DRPTs are at risk for developing melanoma skin cancers. Light treatments offered by a dermatologist can easily remove any worrisome spots that could develop into cancers, but it's still important to know your risk factors and get an annual skin cancer exam.

If you're a DRPT with any of the following factors, you are at higher risk of developing melanoma:

- Light skin
- Light-colored hair
- Sunburn easily
- History of one or more severe sunburns
- Many freckles
- Family members with history of melanoma

While all light-skinned DRPTs should pay heed, any of the above factors will increase your risk. In addition, if you have red hair, your risk *further* increases. Here's why: The MC1R gene is involved in red hair, freckle, and melanoma formation, research reveals. Bottom line? Freckles are not just a cosmetic concern. They may be an early warning sign of the potential for future skin cancers. If you fall into this category, you should be seen by a dermatologist at least annually, especially if you have a history of frequent sunburns. Please consult "The A, B, C, and D of Melanoma" in Chapter Nine for a complete description of what to look out for.

The lip area is most prone to skin cancer because the lips do not secrete sebum, an oil that contains a high concentration of vitamin E, an antioxidant that protects against aging and cancer. That is why many new formulations of Chap Stick and lip balms contain vitamin E to act as a protectant. Health food stores also sell bottles of vitamin E oil. Though it's far too oily for most skin areas, it can be used on the lips with no problem.

## YOUR NEED FOR MOISTURE

Moisturizing is vital to counteract skin dryness. But applying oil in and of itself is not enough. Your goal is to trap water in the skin. That's why I recommend spraying facial water *before* moisturizer application. I'll recommend specific products later in this chapter. Make sure that you apply your moisturizer immediately after spraying the water. If you allow your skin to dry first, it will only increase skin dryness. At the minimum, you should always use a moisturizer with an SPF factor to prevent sun exposure leading to pigmentation. Allow your skin to absorb the product for five minutes before applying your makeup. This will prevent streaking. Foundations can also provide additional moisture and sun protection. Whether or not you opt for a foundation, you may also apply an additional moisturizer, if needed, both morning and evening.

Because your skin is resistant, you need products with ingredients that penetrate the skin, such as retinol and vitamin K, which are contained in many of my recommendations. Products containing alcohol are too drying for you. Study ingredient lists to ensure that any products you are considering purchasing do not contain alcohol among the first seven ingredients. Glycerine, used in many creams, lotions, and soaps, helps to hydrate the skin, so you can look for products that contain it. You'll find information about moisturizing in the next section of this chapter.

**Dr. Baumann's Bottom Line:** My moisturizer recommendations will help your dry skin and reduce the itching and ashiness that often accompany it. Make sure to wear sunscreen to protect your skin and decrease pigmentation.

## Everyday Care for Your Skin Type

The goal of your skin care routine is to address dryness and pigmentation, with products that deliver hydrating, moisturizing, and skin lightening ingredients.

Antioxidants (like vitamins C and E, as well as green tea) can both lessen inflammation leading to dark spots and stave off aging, while retinol has antiaging benefits and can also help to lighten dark spots.

If after two months on the daily regimen, you find that you need more help in addressing skin pigmentation issues, please consult your dermatologist for prescription retiniods.

## DAILY SKIN CARE

---

### STAGE ONE: NONPRESCRIPTION REGIMEN

| AM | PM |
|---|---|
| Step 1: Wash with cleanser | Step 1: Wash with cleanser |
| Step 2: If dark spots are a concern, apply a skin lightener | Step 2: Apply lightener if you have dark spots (optional) |
| Step 3: Spray facial water | Step 3: Spray facial water |
| Step 4: Apply eye cream (optional) | Step 4: Apply eye cream (optional) |
| Step 5: Apply moisturizer with SPF | Step 5: Apply night cream |
| Step 6: Apply foundation with SPF 15 (optional) or use a combination of moisturizer, sunscreen, and foundation to assure a minimum SPF of 15 | |

In the morning, wash your face with a cleanser. If you have dark spots, apply a skin lightener directly to the spots. Next, spray facial water over your entire face and neck, and then, if you wish, apply eye cream. After that, apply a moisturizer that contains SPF. Finally, apply foundation if you wear it.

In the evening, wash with cleanser, and apply a lightener to your dark spots. Next, spray facial water over your entire face and neck, and afterward use eye cream if you wish. Last, apply a night cream.

---

## Cleansers

Cleansers with glycolic acid help your resistant skin absorb other beneficial ingredients delivered in the regimen. They also help brighten your complexion. Glycerin soaps are great for DRPTs, since glycerin is very hydrating. Use any of the many brands available.

## RECOMMENDED CLEANSING PRODUCTS

- $   CeraVe Hydrating Cleanser
- $   Aveeno Positively Radiant Cleanser
- $$  M2 Exfoliating Cleanser
- $$  Nia24 Physical Cleansing Scrub
- $$  Specific Beauty Daily Gentle Cleanser
- $$  Gly Derm Gentle Cleanser 2% (has glycolic acid)
- $$  M.D. Forté Facial Cleanser I, II, or III (has glycolic acid)
- $$  Vivite Exfoliating Facial Cleanser
- $$  Murad Essential-C Cleanser

**Baumann's Choice:** Specific Beauty Daily Gentle Cleanser because it was developed for multi-hued skin tones

## Skin Lighteners

Use a skin lightening gel when you have dark spots. If the products listed below are ineffective, visit a dermatologist to get stronger prescription products.

## RECOMMENDED SKIN LIGHTENERS

- $     Porcelana Skin Discoloration Fade Cream Nighttime Formula
- $     Specific Beauty Skin Brightening Serum
- $$    PCA Skin (pHaze 13) Pigment Gel
- $$    Topix HQS-2 Skin Lightening Cream
- $$    Elure Advanced Whitening Lotion
- $$$   Dr Brandt Flaws No More Lightening Serum
- $$$   SkinCeuticals Phyto +
- $$$   Vivite Vibrance Therapy

**Baumann's Choice:** Vivite Vibrance Therapy is expensive but it works great.

## Facial Waters

Facial waters come from thermal springs and are free of chemicals such as chlorine that are added to our tap water to prevent contamination with algae and other organisms.

Spray water on your face and neck right before applying an eye cream and moisturizer. The moisturizer and eye cream will help trap the water on the skin, giving the skin a reservoir to pull from. This is important when the humidity is low.

## RECOMMENDED FACIAL WATERS

- $ Evian Mineral Water Spray
- $ Avene Thermal Spring Water
- $ La Roche-Posay Thermal Spring Water
- $ Vichy Thermal Spa Water
- $$ Chantecaille Pure Rosewater
- $$ Fresh Rose Marigold Tonic Water
- $$ Shu Uemura Depsea Facial Mist

**Baumann's Choice:** No preference, as they're all good.

## Moisturizers

These moisturizers will help your dry skin and reduce the itching and ashiness that accompany it. In addition, your daytime moisturizer options all contain sun protective factors to help minimize dark spots while preventing skin cancers.

## RECOMMENDED MORNING MOISTURIZERS

- $ Aveeno Positively Radiant Daily Moisturizer SPF 15
- $ RoC Age Diminishing Day Cream SPF 15
- $ Olay Definity Color Recapture SPF 15
- $$ Avon Anew Reversalist Day Renewal Cream SPF 25
- $$ Specific Beauty Daily Hydrating Lotion SPF 30
- $$ Nia24 Sun Damage Prevention Mineral Sunscreen SPF 30
- $$$ SkinCeuticals Daily Moisture (no SPF, so use with a sunscreen or foundation to assure a minimum SPF of 15)

**Baumann's Choice:** Aveeno Positively Radiant Daily Moisturizer SPF 15 because it contains Total Soy Complex that has been proven to even skin tone

## RECOMMENDED EVENING MOISTURIZERS

- $ Aquaglycolic Face Cream
- $ CeraVe Facial Moisturizing Lotion PM
- $ Specific Beauty Night Treatment Complex
- $$ Atopalm MLE Face Cream
- $$ Vivite Night Renewal Facial Cream
- $$ Vichy Nutrilogie 2
- $$ RéVive Moisturizing Renewal Cream with AHA
- $$$ SK-II Skin Refining Treatment
- $$$ Z. Bigatti Re-Storation Enlighten Skin Tone Provider

**Baumann's Choice:** Aquaglycolic Face Cream

## RECOMMENDED EYE CREAMS

- $ Aveeno Ageless Vitality Revitalizing Eye Treatment
- $$ DDF Nutrient K Plus
- $$ Estée Lauder CyberWhite Extra Brightening Eye Cream
- $$ Murad Lighten and Brighten Eye Treatment
- $$$ La Prairie Cellular Eye Moisturizer
- $$$ Sisley Eye and Lip Contour Cream

**Baumann's Choice:** DDF Nutrient K Plus (with vitamin K and horse chestnut)

## Body Moisturizers

Although, in general, body products are outside the scope of this book, your dry skin needs treatment so badly that for you I am making an exception. Heavy creams such as Cetaphil cream and oils such as baby oil are generally not desirable for use on the face because they often feel too greasy. However, you might use one as a night cream, and you can use them on your body. I travel internationally a lot, and I use heavy, greasy creams on the airplane, but I am mortified when I run into someone I know. I usually have on my Gap sweats, no makeup, and a greasy face. Not exactly how I want to be seen!

## RECOMMENDED HEAVY CREAMS
## FOR BODY MOISTURE

$ CeraVe Cream

$ Cetaphil Cream

$ Vaseline Intensive Rescue Moisture Locking Lotion

$ Aveeno Positively Nourishing 24-hour Ultra Hydrating Whipped Soufflé

$$ Ren Mayday Mayday Rescue Balm

$$$ Cle de Peau Beaute Restorative Body Cream

$$$ Laura Mercier Crème Brûlée Soufflé Body Crème

**Baumann's Choice:** CeraVe Cream because it has ceramides

## SHOPPING FOR PRODUCTS

It's a good idea when purchasing skin care products to read labels carefully. Some ingredients will enhance a product's hydrating potential, while others will make your skin drier. If you have a favorite product that contains these ingredients but is not on the list, please enter it at www.skintype solutions.com.

### RECOMMENDED SKIN CARE INGREDIENTS

#### To moisturize and hydrate skin:

- *Ajuga turkestanica*
- Aloe vera
- Borage seed oil
- Canola oil
- Ceramide
- Cholesterol
- Cocoa butter (avoid if you have acne)
- Colloidal oatmeal
- Dexpanthenol (pro-vitamin $B_5$)
- Dimethicone
- Evening primrose oil
- Glycerin
- Jojoba oil
- Lanolin
- Macadamia nut oil
- Olive oil
- Rose hip seed oil
- Safflower oil
- Shea butter

### To get rid of dark spots:

- Arbutin
- Bearberry
- *Cocos nucifera* (coconut fruit juice)
- Cucumber extract
- *Epilobium angustifolium* (willow herb)
- Gallic acid
- *Glycyrrhiza glabra* (licorice extract)
- Hydroquinone
- Kojic acid
- Mulberry
- Niacinamide
- Resorcinol
- Retinol
- Salicylic acid (beta hydroxy acid, or BHA)
- *Saxifraga sarmentosa* extract (strawberry begonia)
- Vitamin C (ascorbic acid)

---

### SKIN CARE INGREDIENTS TO AVOID

### Due to drying:

- Alcohol listed among first seven ingredients
- Cleansers that foam vigorously
- Fragrance

### Due to worsening melasma:

- Estradiol
- Estrogen
- Genistein

## Sun Protection for Your Skin

Your morning moisturizer should contain sunscreen; make sure that your moisturizer, sunscreen, and foundation (whether you use one or more of these products) provide you with a minimum coverage of SPF 15 for normal daily wear. However, if you plan to be in the sun for more than fifteen minutes, apply one of the sunscreen products listed on the following page *over* your moisturizer and under any makeup foundation or powder. (Even if you do this, you should also use a foundation with SPF—you cannot get too much SPF, even if you have dark skin.)

The best sunscreens for you are cream formulations. If you find them too greasy, cover the sunscreen with an SPF-containing powder such as Neutrogena Healthy Defense.

If you have darker skin, you may not like sunscreens containing zinc oxide and titanium dioxide unless they are tinted with color, because they appear so white on the skin. Look for tinted products or those containing micronized zinc (often called Z-cote), an ingredient in SkinCeuticals Ultimate UV Defense SPF 30, which provides protection without the white appearance.

## RECOMMENDED SUN PROTECTION PRODUCTS

$ Aveeno Continuous Protection Sunblock Lotion with SPF 100+ for Face

$ Neutrogena Healthy Defense SPF 30 Daily Moisturizer (comes tinted or untinted)

$$ Solar Protection TIZO3 Translucent Facial Mineral SPF 40 (slightly tinted)

$$ La Roche-Posay Anthelios 60 Ultra Light Sunscreen Fluid for Face

$$ Philosophy When Hope Is Not Enough Age Defense Moisturizer with SPF 20

$$ Replenix CF Advanced Anti-Photoaging Complex SPF 45

$$$ SkinCeuticals Ultimate UV Defense SPF 30 (contains Z-Cote)

**Baumann's Choice:** SkinCeuticals Ultimate UV Defense SPF 30

## Your Makeup

Look for makeup products containing soy, which helps prevent dark spots.

Studies show that vitamin K and substances such as horse chestnut that aid circulation may improve dark circles under the eyes. One eye product containing both vitamin K and horse chestnut is DDF Nutrient K Plus.

## Concealers

You can use a concealer to cover both dark circles under your eyes and dark spots. The following concealers offer a good color selection for those with darker skin tones and are also hydrating rather than drying.

## RECOMMENDED CONCEALERS

$   Mary Kay MK Signature Concealer

$   Neutrogena SkinClearing Concealer

$$   Elizabeth Arden Flawless Finish Sponge-on Cream Makeup

$$   Laura Mercier Secret Concealer

$$   M·A·C Select Cover Up

$$   Dior Skinflash Radiance Booster Pen

$$$   Makeup Forever Professional Full Cover Concealer

$$$   Estée Lauder Re-Nutriv Custom Concealer Duo

**Baumann's Choice:** All of these are good. Select whichever one is a good match for your skin color.


## PROCEDURES FOR YOUR SKIN TYPE

Light-skinned DRPTs can consult a dermatologist for the possible use of lasers, Intense Pulsed Light, and chemical peels to treat their dark spots. Many dermatologists choose to use a combination of these procedures, along with topical bleaching and sunscreen agents. If you have light hair and light skin with lots of freckles, or a history of sunburns, any of these treatments are good for you. You should also see a dermatologist annually to check for skin cancer.

People with darker skin need more careful treatment because any kind of injury or inflammation to the skin can worsen dark spots rather than minimize or eliminate them. For you, a slow approach is best. Most dermatologists choose a regimen of topical prescription medications and chemical peels. If you have dark skin, make sure your dermatologist specializes in treating skin of color and uses only the gentlest procedures.

If you're Asian, your skin appears light-toned, but tends to react similarly to dark-toned skin. Therefore, Asian skin should also be treated very carefully to avoid inflammation and trauma that could worsen the dark spots. So if you are Asian or have a medium skin tone, follow the recommendations for dark skin.

## Light Treatments

Light-skin-toned DRPTs can benefit from light therapy. This procedure lightens dark spots without causing inflammation that leads to more dark spots. Light treatments can also help get rid of redness and blood vessels.

## Chemical Peels

People with darker skin tones or those who do not want (or cannot afford) light treatments can benefit from chemical peels containing glycolic acid, resorcinol, and other depigmenting ingredients. The Jessner's peel is a good choice for this Skin Type. These peels range from $120 to $250 per peel and a series of five to eight is normal.

## ONGOING CARE FOR YOUR SKIN

Sun protection and moisturizing are equally important. Use sunscreen religiously to prevent pigmentation and skin cancer. Unless you have very dark skin, don't forget to get annual checkups to safeguard you from skin cancer, especially if you are a light-skinned or freckled DRPT.

# CHAPTER EIGHTEEN

# Dry, Resistant, Non-Pigmented, and Wrinkled: DRNW

## BAUMANN SKIN TYPE 16

*"My skin was always pretty easy in the summer, but in cold weather the dryness bothers me. Now that I am getting older, the fine lines are showing more and more. I keep hearing about all these expensive antiaging creams with exotic ingredients. I do not know what to buy or who to believe. Which antiaging ingredients really work?"*

## ABOUT YOUR SKIN

The DRNW Skin Type is shared by many Americans. In youth, DRNWs enjoy great skin, with fewer breakouts than the Oily Types; little skin irritation, giving you a wider range of product choices than the sensitive types; and minimal pigmentation to produce the discoloration, dark spots, and freckles that sometimes bother pigmented types. Up until the age of twenty-five, your skin is easy, and most of you don't pay much heed to skin care.

Most people with this Skin Type have light-toned skin and northern European ancestors, with Scandinavian, English, Irish, Scottish, German, Russian, Polish, and other Slavic ethnicities. This delicate pale skin, untouched by freckles or skin discoloration, can be much admired, but it's more fragile than pigmented skin and, unless it's properly cared for, doesn't age that well. This comes as an unpleasant surprise in the second half of life. Currently, baby boomers are reaching this stage, and there's been an explosion of interest in antiaging, skin care, and advanced skin procedures. Is there a connection between the two occurrences? You bet.

Yours is an *overserved* type. Boomers are not the only group interested in these services; adults below the age of forty want to preserve their youthful looks as well. As a result, a plethora of products and services are suddenly appearing in the marketplace, in clinics, and in spas. And while many of them are marketed to DRNWs, unless they are formulated to address your specific combination of the four factors, they may be useless, no matter how pricey they are. How to separate the wheat from the chaff? How to know which products and services are truly effective and which are pretty packaging and marketing hype?

Well, that's my job.

## AN OUNCE OF PREVENTION

For DRNWs in the springtime of life, your skin seems deceptively easy. While other teens fight breakouts, you bask in compliments on your clear, even complexion. Over time, you may experience some dryness, but using any moisturizer brings relief without side effects or reactions. Unlike Sensitive Skin Types (who must avoid irritating ingredients) and Oily Skin Types (who can't bear oil-based sun products), your dry, resistant skin can tolerate most any sunscreen—if you remember to use it.

In youth, your skin is low maintenance, so you neglect simple preventives to assure great skin throughout life. Or you unknowingly abuse your skin, which leads to accelerated aging. And that's why later, in their forties and fifties, the DRNWs come trooping into my office, wanting a last-minute fix.

I urge you, take heed now, because using the right approaches and avoiding the wrong habits will make a big difference long-term. Since young DRNWs, with their "Why worry?" skin, will probably be the least likely to buy this book, give a copy to your DRNW friend, relative, or loved one. You'll be doing her or him a big favor.

## A CLOSE-UP LOOK AT YOUR SKIN

With DRNW skin you may experience any of the following:

- Ease in using sunscreens
- Trouble tanning
- Streaking with self-tanners
- Minimal skin problems in youth, with little or no acne, eczema, skin allergies, or problems with cosmetics or moisturizers
- Crepiness appears around your eyes in your early thirties

- Accelerated wrinkling from mid-thirties on
- Increased dryness and wrinkling in your forties and fifties

Starting young with both sun protection and wrinkle prevention can make a huge difference in how your skin ages. If you follow my instructions, you can wind up looking like a DRNT, especially with the lifestyle factors I'll offer you. Luckily, DRNWs tolerate sunscreens well. Although Oily Types complain that sunscreens feel greasy, DRNWs don't mind it because your dry wrinkle-prone skin needs oil. Instead of tanning, use self-tanners, which provide a safe tanned look, but always use a separate sunscreen as well. Since self-tanners often streak on dry skin, follow my special instructions and recommendations for self-tanner use and products in Chapter Ten, "Self-Tanners." You'll find products that can work for your type in the products section of Chapter Nineteen, following my sunscreen recommendations.

DRNW skin is also more prone to non-melanoma skin cancer, because of several factors:

- Fair-toned skin
- Easily sunburned and hard-to-tan skin
- History of excess sun exposure
- History of smoking
- Diet does not contain enough fruits and vegetables (antioxidants)

According to some estimates, 60 percent of people over the age of forty who meet the above criteria may have at least one incidence of a pre-malignant condition called actinic keratosis. Sixty percent of non-melanoma skin cancers arise from this condition. That's why it's important to know the signs and get checked by a dermatologist annually.

## How to Recognize a Non-Melanoma Skin Cancer

A squamous cell carcinoma (SCC) may appear as red, scaling patches that form scabs in sun-exposed areas such as the face, ears, chest, arms, legs, and back. They don't heal but may be covered by a hard white scale that resembles a wart. Any spot that fits this description and persists for one month or more should be seen by a dermatologist.

A basal cell carcinoma (BCC) may appear as a white, shiny bump, luminous like a pearl. It may have either a central ridge with a little hole or depression, or tiny blood vessels visible in the border. It can also look like a crater or scar that suddenly appears although there has been no prior trauma. Sometimes the border is "ruffled" or heaped up around the central crater.

Enlarged facial oil glands can be easily confused with basal cell carcinoma, since they are both yellowish bumps. Make sure to check out anything suspicious with a dermatologist.

## KEY GUIDELINES FOR YOUR SKIN

Hydration, or keeping moisture in the skin, preserves skin's youthful freshness, so dry types must take special care to hydrate. Drinking lots of water, though possibly helpful for other reasons, will not help skin dehydration. Water is held in the skin by certain lipids, or fats, which is why I recommend that you consume healthy omega-3 fats (obtainable from supplements and foods such as flaxseed and salmon). Skin damage and aging occur through the formation of free radicals, renegade molecules that break down the basic skin biochemicals that maintain skin structure and safeguard hydration. Free radicals promote the dissolution of collagen, hyaluronic acid, and elastin, the three cornerstones of youthful skin. Antioxidants quench free radicals to protect these vital skin chemicals.

Antioxidants can be obtained from foods and supplements, and via topical skin products. DRNWs under the age of thirty should seek out skin products that contain antioxidants like vitamins C and E, green tea, coenzyme $Q_{10}$, and Argan Oil (often found in moisturizers appropriate for this type, such as Josie Maran Argan Oil). In your thirties, I suggest starting a prescription retinoid—with the caution that pregnant women and nursing mothers, as well as those who plan to become pregnant, should defer retinoid use from the time you plan to become pregnant until after you've finished breastfeeding. At the first sign of wrinkles, add an alpha hydroxy acid or polyhydroxy acid to your regimen. You can find my recommendations later in this chapter. DRNWs of all ages should use a daily sunscreen. For more information about preventing wrinkles, please consult Chapter Two, pages 23 and 24.

Menopause can be a hard time for DRNW women. Falling estrogen levels can dry out—and thin out—your skin. In fact, studies have shown a sharp decline in skin thickness in women after the fifth decade of life. Most declines in skin collagen, a key factor in skin thickness, occur during the first few years after menopause, with a 30 percent decline in the first five years, and an average decline of 2.1 percent per postmenopausal year thereafter over a period of twenty years. Hormone replacement therapy or the use of topical estrogen reverses this process, many studies show. However, given other concerns about HRT, this is a decision you will want to make with your primary care physician.

## CHOOSING THE RIGHT MOISTURIZER

There are thousands of moisturizers, antiaging creams, and treatments to prevent wrinkling, and they are all targeted to you. Unlike your close Skin Type cousins, the DRPWs, who are underserved, you're one of the largest market segments. Companies are trying to help you—and going after your dollar. The upside? You have so many options. The downside? You have so many options, but no way of knowing what really works. That's why it's important to learn what kinds of products and ingredients are of real benefit.

You can get temporary relief from dryness and wrinkles with many different products as many moisturizers hydrate and plump up the skin, making fine lines disappear for anywhere from an hour to two days.

But I'll let you in on a little trade secret. Companies asserting their product reduces wrinkles in a certain number of days often base these claims on in-house studies, designed so that the participants use no moisturizer for a week prior to the study. As a result, dry types will develop tiny dry lines especially around the eyes, visible in photos taken at their first visit, where the "baseline" condition of their skin is documented prior to use of the product. Then they use the study cream and what do you know? Those fine lines appear minimized after a few days of moisturizing.

While no over-the-counter creams have been convincingly proven to improve wrinkles long-term, your dry skin requires regular moisturizing, so why not minimize the appearance of wrinkles as well? Your resistant skin can tolerate a higher concentration of active ingredients than some other types. However, not everything you put on your face can be absorbed and utilized as you intend.

## EVERYDAY CARE FOR YOUR SKIN TYPE

You will age more gracefully if you are proactive in maintaining and protecting your skin in youth. And it's never too late to start. With medical advances happening every day, who knows what the average life span will be? Take action now so you can continue looking your best, even if you live to be 150.

The goal of your skin care routine is to address dryness and wrinkles with products that deliver antioxidants, moisturizers, and retinoids.

## DAILY SKIN CARE

### REGIMEN

| AM | PM |
|---|---|
| Step 1: Wash with cleanser containing glycolic acid | Step 1: Wash with cleanser containing glycolic acid |
| Step 2: Apply antioxidant serum | Step 2: Apply antioxidant serum |
| Step 3: Spray facial water | Step 3: Spray facial water |
| Step 4: Apply eye cream | Step 4: Apply eye cream |
| Step 5: Apply moisturizer with SPF, assuring that your combination of moisturizer and sunscreen provides a minimum SPF of 15 | Step 5: Apply night cream |

In the morning, wash your face with cleanser, then apply an antioxidant serum. Spray facial water on your face and neck, then immediately apply eye cream and a moisturizer containing sunscreen.

In the evening, wash with the same cleanser, then apply antioxidant serum. Then spray facial water, next apply eye cream and nighttime moisturizer. If you are over thirty, choose a night cream with retinol, alpha hydroxy acids, or vitamin C. Or consult a dermatologist for a prescription retinoid.

## Cleansers

Never wash your face with soap or shampoo, as any products that foam contain detergent that is much too drying for your skin. Instead use cleansers that contain alpha hydroxy acids, such as glycolic acid and lactic acid, which help hydrate the skin and increase collagen production. In addition, they remove the top layer of dead skin cells so that beneficial ingredients can penetrate. In this regimen, after cleansing, you'll be using antioxidant serums, which will act more powerfully when they follow these AHAs. Some of my recommendations don't contain AHAs for those who prefer not to use them. They can make you sun sensitive, so those of you who don't wear sunscreen may choose a non-AHA cleanser.

## RECOMMENDED CLEANSERS

$   Aqua Glycolic Facial Cleanser

$   Aveeno Positively Ageless Daily Exfoliating Cleanser

$   Glycolix Elite Moisturizing Cleanser

$$   Vivite Replenish Hydrating Facial Cleanser

$$   M.D. Forté Facial Cleanser II (with glycolic acid 15%)

$$   M.D. Forté Facial Cleanser III (with glycolic acid 20%)

$$   Murad Essential-C Cleanser (with antioxidants, vitamin C, and phospholipids)

$$   iS Clinical Cleansing Complex

$$   Vichy Rich Detoxifying Cleansing Milk

$$$   Nia24 Gentle Cleansing Cream

$$$   Jurlique Balancing Cleansing Lotion

$$$   N.V. Perricone M.D. Olive Oil Polyphenols Gentle Cleanser with DMAE

$$$   Elizabeth Arden Millenium Hydrating Cleanser

**Baumann's Choice:** M.D. Forté Facial Cleanser II and then progress to III after one month.

## Antioxidant Serums

Serums are a good way to deliver the concentrated antioxidants your type needs for wrinkle treatment and prevention. My choice here, SkinCeuticals C + E, has the right vitamin C at the right pH and is packaged properly. The research on this product is stellar. It's expensive, but its benefits give you a reason to splurge. If you plan to have sun exposure against my advice, you should choose the SkinCeuticals C & E Ferulic serum, which may help prevent some of the sun's damage to your skin.

### RECOMMENDED ANTIOXIDANT SERUMS

$$   Olay Pro X Skin Tightening Serum

$$   SoPhyto MultiVitamin Skin Drops

$$   Josie Maran Argan Oil

$$   Replenix Power of 3 Cream

$$$   Boske Dermaceuticals Alchemist C (Normal to Dry)

$$$   Combray by Solenne

$$$   iS Clinical Super Serum Advance

$$$   SkinCeuticals C & E Ferulic

**Baumann's Choice:** SkinCeuticals C & E Ferulic or iS Clinical Super Serum Advance

## Facial Water

DRNWs should avoid toners, which often contain drying alcohol. Instead, use a facial water. Spray it on your face immediately before you apply moisturizer. The moisturizer helps trap the water on the skin, giving the skin a reservoir to pull from. Note that although you may like the "soothing" ingredients in the more expensive of these products, you don't actually need them.

### RECOMMENDED FACIAL WATERS

- $ Evian Mineral Water Spray
- $ Twinlab Na-Pca Spray with Aloe Vera
- $ La Roche-Posay Thermal Spring Water
- $$ Shu Uemura Depsea Facial Mist
- $$ Vichy Thermal Spa Water

**Baumann's Choice:** Twinlab Na-Pca Spray with Aloe Vera because it may help to protect your skin barrier

## Moisturizers

If you are under thirty, look for moisturizers containing antioxidants. If you are older, you will need heavier moisturizers. Those over thirty should also look for a nighttime moisturizer that contains retinol.

In some situations you may want to use a lighter moisturizer. Before a big evening event, I suggest using a facial scrub followed by a hydrating mask (see the "Exfoliation" and "Masks" sections of this chapter). Once the mask is removed, apply a thin layer of light moisturizer followed by your evening makeup. (Not too much moisturizer. You do not want to look shiny.) Your face will look fresh and flake-free. One good option is Caudalíe Anti-Wrinkle Ultra Nourishing Cream. Lacking sunscreen, it's not good for daytime use, and it's too light for nighttime use, but it works in this case.

## RECOMMENDED DAYTIME MOISTURIZERS (WITH SPF)

$ Boots No7 Protect & Perfect Day Cream SPF 15

$ Purpose Dual Treatment Moisture Lotion with SPF 15

$$ Prevage Day Ultra Protection Anti-Aging Moisturizer SPF 30

$$ Estée Lauder Daywear Plus Multi Protection Anti-Oxidant Creme SPF 15 for Dry Skin

$$ Exuviance Essential Multi-Defense Day Creme SPF 15

$$ RevaléSkin CoffeeBerry Day Cream

**Baumann's Choice:** Estée Lauder Daywear Plus Multi Protection Anti-Oxidant Creme

## RECOMMENDED NIGHTTIME MOISTURIZERS

$ Burt's Bees Carrot Nutritive Night Crème

$ Olay Total Effects Night Firming Cream

$ Neutrogena Clinical Facial Lifting Wrinkle Treatment

$ Aveeno Positively Ageless Lifting and Firming Daily Moisturizer SPF 30

$$ Atopalm MLE Face Cream

$$ Exuviance Evening Restorative Complex

$$ Vivite Night Renewal Facial Cream

$$ Kiehl's Açaí Damage-Correcting Moisturizer

$$ Korres Quercetin and Oak Age-Reversing Night Cream

$$ Sophyto Mega Omegas Day Face Moisturiser

$$ Shu Uemura Depsea Hydrability Moisturizing Cream

$$$ Fresh Elixir Ancien Face Treatment Oil

$$$ Caudalíe Anti-Wrinkle Ultra Nourishing Cream

$$$ Sisley Paris Comfort Extreme Night Skin Care

$$$ SK-II Skin Signature Melting Rich Cream

**Baumann's Choice:** I like Atopalm if your skin is parched and Sophyto Mega Omegas Day Face Moisturiser if you want something organic.

## RECOMMENDED EVENING MOISTURIZERS WITH RETINOL

$ RoC Retinol Correxion Deep Wrinkle Night Cream

$ Neutrogena Healthy Skin Anti-Wrinkle Cream Original Formula

$$ Topix Replenix Retinol Plus Smoothing Serum 2x

$$ Topix Replenix Retinol Plus Smoothing Serum 5x
$$ PCA Skin Retinol Renewal
$$ Philosophy Help Me Face Cream

**Baumann's Choice:** I like all the ones in the $$ range.

### RECOMMENDED EYE CREAMS

$ Neutrogena Radiance Boost Eye Cream
$ Nivea Visage Coenzyme $Q_{10}$ Plus Wrinkle Control Eye Cream
with SPF 4
$$ Caudalíe w/ Pulpe Vitaminee Eye and Lip Cream
$$ Dr. Brandt Lineless Eye Cream
$$ Elizabeth Arden Prevage Anti-Aging Eye Treatment
$$$ Kate Somerville Line Release Under Eye Repair Cream
$$$ SK-II Signs Eye Cream

**Baumann's Choice:** Elizabeth Arden Prevage Anti-Aging Eye Treatment with Idebenone

## Moisture Emergency

During travel, when engaged in winter sports, in dry climates, or other extreme dry conditions, dry types may have what I call a "moisture emergency," when more intensive moisturizing is required. If your skin is excessively dry, cracked, or in need of moisture, you can use these heavier products, which can also be applied to your feet, hands, or body. Although a little greasy, they're formulated for problematic dryness and definitely come in handy from time to time. Since they are right in between prescription medications and regular moisturizers, you may have to ask your pharmacist for them, as they are not usually displayed with regular moisture creams.

### RECOMMENDED HEAVY MOISTURIZERS FOR FACE OR BODY

$ Cetaphil Moisturizing Cream (better for body than face)
$$ Aveeno Advanced Care Moisturizing Cream
$$ CeraVe Cream
$$ Elizabeth Arden Eight Hour Cream Skin Protectant
$$ Philosophy When Hope Is Not Enough Omega 3·6·9
Replenishing Body Lotion

$$ Osmotics TriCeram
$$$ Korres Bitter Almond Body Milk

**Baumann's Choice:** Atopalm is the least greasy and best for facial use. Aveeno Advanced Care Moisturizing Cream is my favorite for body use.

## Exfoliation

You should exfoliate once or twice a week, unless you are on retinoids. When using a retinoid, you don't need to exfoliate unless you'd like to remove superficial scaling caused by the retinoid. In that case, you can exfoliate once a week.

### RECOMMENDED SCRUBS

$ Aveeno Active Naturals Skin Brightening Daily Scrub
$ Nivea for Men Deep Cleaning Face Scrub
$ St. Ives Swiss Formula Invigorating Apricot Scrub
$$ Clinique 7 Day Scrub Cream
$$ Elemis Skin Buff
$$ L'Occitane Brightening Smoothing Exfoliator
$$ Vivite Exfoliating Facial Cleanser
$$ Philosophy The Microdelivery Mini Peel Pads
$$$ Dr. Brandt Microdermabrasion in a Jar
$$$ Clarisonic Mia Sonic Skin Cleansing System

**Baumann's Choice:** Clinique 7 Day Scrub Cream. I love the texture and the moisture it leaves behind.

## Masks

Once or twice a week, you might like to use a hydrating mask. My choice here is the least expensive product, because I would rather see you spend your money on a prescription retinoid and an expensive serum. Masks are not that important, anyway; they don't stay on your face very long.

If you are not trying to save money, use the Caudalíe mask. It has grape seed extract, which will give your skin some wrinkle prevention, and it's very luxurious.

## RECOMMENDED MASKS

$   Vitalic Pomegranate Mask 6-pack
$$   Fresh Rose Face Mask
$$   Laura Mercier Intensive Moisture Mask
$$$   Caudalíe Moisturizing Cream Mask
$$$   Lancôme Hydra-Intense Masque

**Baumann's Choice:** Caudalíe Moisturizing Cream Mask

## SHOPPING FOR PRODUCTS

When you purchase products, be sure to read ingredient labels carefully. With your resistant skin, the only ingredients you need to avoid are the detergents in cleansers and shampoos. But you can also look for ingredients that help treat dryness and prevent wrinkles. If you have favorite products that contain these ingredients but are not on my lists, please share them with me at www.skintypesolutions.com.

---

### RECOMMENDED SKIN CARE INGREDIENTS

#### *To prevent wrinkles:*

- Basil
- Caffeine
- *Camilla sinensis* (green tea, white tea)
- Carrot extract
- Coenzyme $Q_{10}$ (ubiquinone)
- Copper peptide
- Curcumin (tetra-hydracurcumin or turmeric)
- Ferulic acid
- Feverfew
- Genistein (soy)
- Ginger
- Ginseng
- Grape seed extract
- Idebenone
- Lutein
- Lycopene
- Phytol
- *Punica granatum* (pomegranate)
- Pycnogenol (a pine bark extract)
- Rosemary
- Silymarin
- Yucca

### To improve the appearance of wrinkles:

- Alpha hydroxy acids
- Citric acid
- Gluconolactone
- Glycolic acid
- Lactic acid
- Phytic acid
- Polyhydroxy acids
- Retinol

### To hydrate and moisturize skin:

- *Ajuga turkestanica*
- Aloe vera
- Apricot kernel oil
- Borage seed oil
- Canola oil
- Ceramide
- Cholesterol
- Cocoa butter
- Colloidal oatmeal
- Dexpanthenol (pro-vitamin $B_5$)
- Dimethicone
- Evening primrose oil
- Glycerin
- Jojoba oil
- Macadamia nut oil
- Olive oil
- Safflower oil
- Shea butter

**SKIN CARE INGREDIENTS TO AVOID**

### Due to drying:

- Detergents that foam vigorously. A little foam is acceptable if you have a higher O/D score, such as 17–26, but nonfoaming cleansers are best if your O/D score is under 17.

## Sun Protection for Your Skin

It's essential that you wear sunscreen every day. If you don't expect more than fifteen minutes of exposure, you can use a daytime moisturizer or foundation that contains SPF. But if you plan to be in the sun for more than fifteen minutes, layer another sunscreen on top of your moisturizer and under your foundation. Make sure that whether you use one or multiple products, you obtain a minimum coverage of SPF 15. For more than one hour of sun exposure, reapply sunscreen every hour and use an SPF of at least 30. When you swim, use a waterproof sunscreen and reapply after immersion.

Creams are best for your type. Use a broad-spectrum sunscreen that covers both UVA and UVB.

### RECOMMENDED SUN PROTECTION PRODUCTS

- $ Aveeno Continuous Protection Sunblock Lotion SPF 30 or SPF 45
- $ Eucerin Sensitive Facial Skin Extra Protective Moisture Lotion with SPF 30
- $ Blue Lizard Australian Suncream SPF 30 Baby
- $$ Topix Citrix Antioxidant Cleanser
- $$ Dermalogica Solar Defense Booster SPF 30
- $$ Prevage Day Ultra Protection Anti-Aging Moisturizer SPF 30
- $$ La Roche-Posay Anthelios SX SPF 15 Cream
- $$ Nia24 Sun Damage Prevention 100% Mineral Sunscreen
- $$$ Lancôme Rénergie Intense Lift SPF 15
- $$$ Orlane Anti-Wrinkle Sun Cream for the Face SPF 15

**Baumann's Choice:** Aveeno Continuous Protection Sunblock Lotion SPF 30 or SPF 45

## Your Makeup

In choosing a foundation be sure to use one that contains oil. An oil-free foundation is not right for your dry skin. When possible, use a foundation that contains SPF.

### RECOMMENDED FOUNDATIONS

- $ Neutrogena Healthy Skin Liquid Makeup SPF 20
- $ Revlon Age Defying Makeup
- $$ Dr. Hauschka Translucent Makeup
- $$ Elizabeth Arden Ceramide Plump Perfect Makeup SPF 15
- $$ Laura Mercier Moisturizing Foundation
- $$ M·A·C Studio Fix Fluid SPF 25
- $$$ Chantecaille Real Skin Foundation SPF 30 for Dry Skin
- $$$ Guerlain Parure Aqua Radiant Feel-Good Foundation

**Baumann's Choice:** Laura Mercier Moisturizing Foundation

## PROCEDURES FOR YOUR SKIN TYPE

Along with prescription medications, botulinum toxin injections and dermal fillers are mainstays for treating wrinkles for your Skin Type.

For light-skinned DRNWs, dermabrasion will help treat deep wrinkles. In addition, procedures such as Titan, Thermage, and Ulthera treat aging skin. Ask your dermatologist for more information.

## ONGOING CARE FOR YOUR SKIN

Avoid the sun and stop smoking to preserve your skin. Plus, use retinols and retinoids to reverse sun damage and the signs of aging. Eat an antioxidant-rich diet. If your pocketbook will permit, go for procedures that will bring real results. Your resistant, non-pigmented skin will help protect you from the side effects that other Skin Types develop after these procedures. The latest technology is there for you.

# CHAPTER NINETEEN

# Dry, Resistant, Non-Pigmented, and Tight: DRNT

## BAUMANN SKIN TYPE 14

■

*"I do not have any difficult skin issues except dryness. I am under forty years old but I am interested in keeping my skin looking its best. Is a moisturizer alone enough for me?"*

### ABOUT YOUR SKIN

Congratulations. You won the Skin Type lottery. You have dream skin. You've probably never been near a dermatologist's office. In your teens and twenties, you were the envy of all your friends because you had the best skin—minimal acne, no oiliness, few freckles. Perhaps you suffered from occasional dry skin patches, but this was no big deal. If you are older, you may have noticed that your skin has become drier, but you can control dryness with most moisturizers. If you're older than forty-five, and not taking hormones, your skin's dryness may have worsened due to the loss of estrogen. But you still look pretty good, and people often guess your age at five to ten years younger than you actually are.

When it comes to skin care, the DRNT's motto is "Feel good, look good." You don't realize how lucky you are to have low-maintenance DRNT skin. When others compliment your skin, you have no idea what they mean. It's just skin, isn't it? You're particularly lucky if you have a darker skin tone because you have the benefits of darker skin without the dark spots and patches that sometimes plague a related but pigmented skin type, the DRPT.

You're more concerned with how you feel than with how you look.

Although you don't differentiate skin care from overall self-care, you do treat yourself right by eating a healthy diet and getting plenty of rest and exercise. Many people with this Skin Type value quality of life and make choices that maintain it.

A W/T score always results from a combination of genes and lifestyle choices. A light-skinned, dry, non-pigmented type is prone to sun damage, and if you'd persisted in tanning your non-tannable skin (or repeatedly burned and tanned), then you'd most likely be a DRNW rather than a DRNT. If you have dark skin, the melanin in your skin helps protect you from wrinkles and skin cancer. Other factors also help keep you a T Skin Type, such as having T ancestors, eating a lot of antioxidant-filled fruits and vegetables, ceasing smoking, avoiding secondhand smoke, and maintaining a steady slender weight, rather than going through yo-yo weight gain and loss, which stretches the skin. Stress contributes to the body's inflammatory response, one factor in skin sensitivity. Like everyone, you experience stress, but you've found ways to cope.

## DRNTs AND LIFESTYLE CHOICES

How do DRNTs luck out in the Skin Type lottery? They often preserve their skin through good habits, such as eating a skin-healthy diet and taking beneficial supplements like omega-3 fats. Many try relaxation therapies, like Reiki or massage, or go to spas. Pampering their dry skin, health-conscious DRNTs often avoid sun exposure or use protective sunscreens. Unlike sensitive types, who are irritated by many sunscreen ingredients, DRNTs can use anything from Coppertone to Aubrey's to a high-end brand. As a result, it's easier to use sunscreen consistently to protect from the sun's harsh rays. Moderating stress through exercise, like walking or yoga, or lifestyle behaviors, like meditation or journaling, helps them maintain balance in this challenging modern world. While some greet stress by going into overdrive, DRNTs tend to slow down, set priorities, and set boundaries.

## DRNTs AND SKIN COLOR

The majority of DRNTs have light to medium skin tones, while dark-skin-toned DRNTs are in the minority. Most people with dark skin are pigmented types because they have higher pigment levels overall than light-skin toned people. However, the questionnaire differentiates between overall pigment levels and pigment problems, such as melasma or dark spots. Therefore, dark-toned DRNTs will be free of the dark spots that trouble many people of color. They owe their smooth, even skin to a combination of lucky genes and sun avoidance. Dark-skinned DRNTs typically have different sun habits than the majority of people of color. Most dark-skinned people assume that they don't need sunscreen but sun exposure can increase pigmentation, resulting in an uneven complexion. In contrast to other people of color, I've noticed that dark-skinned DRNTs *do* use sunscreen or they avoid the sun. As a result, like the stunning fashion model Iman, they have exceptionally even complexions. What good fortune. Moreover, although light-skin-toned DRNTs are at higher risk for skin cancer, dark-skin-toned DRNTs are protected by their overall pigment levels—the best of all possible worlds.

## CLOSE-UP LOOK AT YOUR SKIN

With DRNT skin you may experience any of the following:

- Few noticeable skin problems
- Even-toned skin
- Ease in using a wide range of skin products
- Few breakouts, if any
- Inability to tan
- High susceptibility to sunburn, especially after swimming
- Streaking with self-tanners
- Normal to dry skin in youth
- Dryness worsens for women at perimenopause and menopause
- Noticeable dryness after bathing or swimming
- Increased risk of non-melanoma skin cancers

Truthfully, I don't know how many people have this Skin Type, since DRNTs rarely consult a dermatologist unless they develop a skin disease such as psoriasis or skin cancer. Unfortunately, light-skinned DRNTs may be at a high risk of skin cancer. Since you have trouble tanning, you're more likely to abuse your skin in youth by submitting to excess sun exposure or even ultraviolet tanning beds. If you bypassed that temptation, good for you. You will likely have a lifetime of great, albeit a little dry, skin. All you have to do is moisturize, use sun protection, and enjoy your luck.

On the other hand, if gardening, tennis, fishing, golf, or other outdoor activities exposed you to frequent and unprotected sun, and you have light skin color, make sure to go for an annual skin exam to rule out skin cancer.

Your lack of pigmentation may set you up for it, the light-skinned DRNT's most significant downside. Please see Chapter Seven, "How to Recognize a Non-Melanoma Skin Cancer," for guidelines on how to detect it so that you can also make a special trip if you develop anything that looks suspicious. Also, schedule annual checkups with your dermatologist to monitor your skin.

## EFFECTIVE SELF-TANNING

DRNTs often have trouble achieving a smooth tan with a self-tanner, but I can help you get better results. All tanners, both spray and rub-on products, contain the same chemical, dihydroxyacetone, which chemically reacts with acids in the topmost level of the skin cells. The surface of dry skin consists of many dead skin cells, invisible to the naked eye (but visible under a microscope), which collect in heaps and valleys. These cells contain proteins that react to the dihydroxyacetone by turning an orange-brown color. As a result, areas with a thicker layer of dead cells will appear darker than where cells are thinner. The self-tan will therefore look spotty.

An exfoliating scrub, used prior to self-tanner application, will remove the heaped-up skin cells, creating an even surface to permit a more consistent tan. Although this exfoliation is ideal for everyone, it's especially important for Dry Skin Types. I'll therefore be recommending self-tanners and exfoliation products in a later section of this chapter.

## DRYNESS IN DARK-COLORED SKIN

Dark-skin-toned DRNTs have the even complexion of non-pigmented skin along with the skin cancer protection of pigmented skin. But dark-toned DRNT skin does have one downside, dryness.

Many dark-skin-toned DRNTs do not use daily sunscreen because spots and wrinkles aren't a problem. However, even dark-skin-toned people can benefit from daily sunscreen application.

With dark DRNT skin you may experience any of the following:

- Even-toned facial skin
- Ease in using a wide range of skin products
- Dry, rough skin with an ashy tone
- Darkness over knees, elbows, and knuckles

- Itching
- Increased dryness after bathing or swimming
- Sunscreens appear whitish or violet on your skin

Ashiness (a grayish skin tone) can be worsened by anything that dries out the skin, such as detergents, harsh hair chemicals, hotel soaps, wind, or cold weather. In people with darker-toned skin, ashiness occurs because the superficial layer of the skin becomes flaky and white while the underlying dark skin peeks through. To solve this common complaint among dark-skin-toned DRNTs, moisturize. A number of fine products are marketed specifically for this condition, such as Aveeno Daily Moisturizing Lotion with Natural Colloidal Oatmeal. Avoiding harsh soaps, such as hotel soaps, will help prevent this condition.

## YOUR PRODUCT OPTIONS

Your skin is easy. You can use whatever you choose. Some of you prefer expensive brands because you attribute your excellent skin condition to their supposedly high-quality ingredients, while others reach for whatever's available. In many instances, the difference between the high- and low-end products is not as great as people believe, and the cheaper ones can be better for your skin. It all comes down to the right ingredients for a given type.

You have less need to seek out specialized ingredients and products (or avoid bothersome ones) than many other types. Beyond basic cleansing, your only real need is moisturizing.

When it comes to shopping for products, some DRNTs will stay loyal to products they like, while others experiment with new products they find appealing due to their packaging, color, scent, or some other association. DRNTs don't need prescription products. Old-fashioned glycerin and rose water, a classic skin-hydration product, was good enough for your grandmother and can be good enough for you. Unlike sensitive types, who may react to perfumes in products, you can benefit from products with mild essential oils such as lavender, chamomile, and rose.

## DRNTs AND WATER

Although many health books suggest drinking water to increase skin hydration, what you drink does not impact your skin's ability to hold on to water. Poor hydration is due to damage to the skin barrier, and drinking water makes no difference. Cells on the surface of the skin line up to form what is called the skin barrier. These cells look something like a row of bricks in a wall held together by mortar. When the mortar breaks down or weakens, the wall cannot hold, and the skin cells (acting like bricks) move and leave gaps. As a result, skin cannot hold water *in* the skin to maintain the skin's cellular integrity.

All dry types need to hydrate the skin, but this is easier for dry, resistant types, like you. Resistant skin gives you a more solid skin barrier, but you will still need to preserve and hydrate it, more than oily types. Increase the skin's ability to hold moisture with the skin care I'll recommend.

Interestingly, water immersion *decreases* the water content of the skin. Long baths, lap swimming, or ocean sports (like snorkeling or scuba diving) that involve soaking in the water over an extended time period are harmful to your skin. First of all, research indicates that prolonged water exposure of any kind can dehydrate skin by undermining its ability to retain water. Chlorinated water, commonly found in swimming pools, is especially dehydrating. Hot water and hard water (which contains more calcium) are also rougher on the skin. For this reason, dermatologists usually suggest that dry types take a quick bath or shower (five to ten minutes) in lukewarm water. After bathing, use a soft—not rough—towel to gently pat the skin partially dry. Apply a moisturizer immediately afterward while the skin is still damp. The oil in the moisturizer helps trap the water on the skin surface and helps the skin to absorb it.

## DRNTs AND DRYNESS

To minimize skin dryness, what you wear may be as important as the skin care products you use. Studies show that with dry skin, people are more sensitive to fabric roughness than when the skin is well hydrated. DRNTs and other dry types may feel irritated and uncomfortable wearing wool and other rough fabrics. Certain fabrics, like rough linen or polyester, may actually worsen dry skin and lead to ashiness. Wearing softer fabrics or using fabric softeners may help.

Whether it's skin care, hair care, or household cleansing products, avoid anything that foams, since foaming products contain detergents. Detergents from soaps, shampoos, cleansing products and laundry detergents can increase dryness. Use non-foaming skin and hair care products. Wear gloves when washing dishes or cleaning. In laundering, use less soap and assure that it's rinsed thoroughly from clothing, bedding, towels, and other fabrics that come into contact with your skin. In addition, in certain instances, chemicals used in dry cleaning can irritate the skin. The chemicals used by ecological dry cleaners may be easier to tolerate.

## YOUR SKIN TYPE'S SOLUTION

Moisturizing is essential both in youth, to safeguard your skin's natural moisture, and as you age, to minimize progressive dryness. For your daily skin care, use a moisturizer for daytime and a second, richer product for nighttime. You can use almost any product without a problem. However, to avoid hyped products of little real benefit, choose the most effective moisturizers by learning about the key ingredients you need.

There are two main categories of moisturizers: occlusives and humectants. Some ingredients belong to both categories. Occlusives "occlude" the skin, which means they prevent water from evaporating. Plastic wrap such as Saran Wrap, which protects food by keeping it hydrated, acts in exactly the same way. Common occlusive ingredients include petrolatum (as in petroleum jelly), most types of oil (such as sesame, mineral, and olive oil), propylene glycol (a popular additive in cosmetics), and dimethicone (a silicone derivative).

Humectants, such as glycerin and hyaluronic acid, act differently from occlusives. Due to their high water-absorption capabilities, humectants draw water *into* the skin. However, humectants can also act as turncoats because their water-drawing action is unidirectional. Here's how that works: Although they usually draw water *from* the environment *into* the skin to hydrate it, in low-humidity conditions, that action is reversed. Instead, they may take water *from* the skin (often from the deeper epidermis and dermis) and send it out. This results in increased skin dryness. For this reason, they work better when combined with occlusives. For DRNTs, the best moisturizers contain combinations of both occlusive and humectant ingredients.

**Dr. Baumann's Bottom Line:** As a DRNT, you should avoid prolonged bathing and rough fabrics, use non-foaming, soap-free cleansers, and moisturize frequently. If you have light skin, make sure to wear sunscreen and get annual checkups to detect skin cancer.

## EVERYDAY CARE FOR YOUR SKIN

The goal of your skin care routine is to address dryness and ashy skin with products that deliver occlusive and humectant moisturizing ingredients.

Your skin care needs are simple: Moisturize, moisturize, moisturize. With your resistant skin, you can use almost any product. However, follow my recommendations below to find the most effective moisturizers, which combine occlusives and humectants.

You don't need any prescription medications; you are one of the few groups for whom I do not recommend a retinoid—it's too drying.

### DAILY SKIN CARE

---

### REGIMEN

| AM | PM |
|---|---|
| Step 1: Wash with creamy non-foaming cleanser or cleansing oil | Step 1: Wash with same cleanser as in AM |
| Step 2: Apply eye cream (optional) | Step 2: Spray facial water |
| Step 3: Apply daytime moisturizer with SPF, assuring that your combination of moisturizer, sunscreen, and foundation delivers an SPF of at least 15 | Step 3: Apply eye cream (optional) |
| Step 4: Apply a foundation with SPF (optional) | Step 4: Apply nighttime moisturizer |

In the morning, wash with a creamy non-foaming cleanser or a cleansing oil. Because your skin is tight, eye cream is not a must for you, but if you wish, apply eye cream next. Then apply a daytime moisturizer that contains SPF. Finish with a foundation that also contains SPF if you wish to wear one.

In the evening, wash with the same cleanser you used in the morning. Spray facial water, then apply eye cream if you choose to. Last, apply a nighttime moisturizer.

---

## Cleansers

Because your skin is dry, you should stay away from any soaps or cleansers that foam vigorously. Use a cream cleanser or a cold cream instead.

Did you know that using oil to cleanse the skin is quite popular in Asia? This is actually a great idea for very Dry Skin Types. Below I've listed some of my favorites cleansers, including Shu Uemura, which offers a "collector's edition" of its Skin Purifying oils in adorable bottles.

### RECOMMENDED CLEANSERS

- $ CeraVe Cleanser
- $ Aveeno Skin Brightening Daily Scrub
- $$ Caudalíe Gentle Cleanser
- $$ Topix Glycolix Elite 10% Moisturizing Cleanser
- $$ Estée Lauder Soft Clean Tender Creme Cleanser
- $$ Origins Pure Cream Cleanser
- $$ Nia24 Gentle Cleanser
- $$ SoPhyto Ultra Mild Silken Cleanser
- $$ Kate Somerville Gentle Daily Wash
- $$$ Jo Malone Avocado Cleansing Milk
- $$$ Prada Purifying Milk/Face

**Baumann's Choice:** CeraVe Cleanser

### RECOMMENDED CLEANSING OILS

- $ Jojoba Cleansing Oil
- $$ Shu Uemura High Performance Balancing Cleansing Oil Enriched
- $$ SK II Facial Treatment Cleansing Oil
- $$$ Decléor Cleansing Oil
- $$$ Seikisho Cleansing Oil

**Baumann's Choice:** Shu Uemura High Performance Balancing Cleansing Oil Enriched

## Facial Water

A DRNT should *never* use a toner.

Spraying your skin with a facial water prior to moisturizing can help hydrate it. Many moisturizers contain humectants that pull water from the atmosphere. If you use a humectant in a low-humidity environment, such as in an airplane, it can pull water from your skin rather than the environment. Spraying a facial water on your skin before applying a moisturizer will give the humectant water to pull *into* the skin rather than the other way around.

## RECOMMENDED FACIAL WATERS

- $ Evian Mineral Water Spray
- $ La Roche-Posay Thermal Spring Water
- $ Vichy Thermal Spring Water
- $$ Avène Thermal Water Spray
- $$ Shu Uemura Depsea Facial Mist
- $$$ Jurlique Recovery Mist MD (Moisture Depleted)

**Baumann's Choice:** Evian is the least expensive and easiest to find.

## Moisturizers

The best moisturizers contain both occlusive and humectant ingredients. You should find and regularly use two good moisturizers. The one for daytime use should contain sunscreen, while your nighttime moisturizer can be richer.

## RECOMMENDED MORNING MOISTURIZERS
### (WITH SUNSCREEN)

- $ Aveeno Positively Ageless Daily Moisturizer SPF 30
- $ Eucerin Q10 Anti-Wrinkle Sensitive Skin Lotion SPF 15
- $ La Roche-Posay Anthelios SX Daily Moisturizing Sunscreen with Mexoryl, SPF 15
- $ Specific Beauty Daily Hydrating Lotion with SPF 30
- $$ Clinique Superdefense SPF 25 Age Defense Moisturizer
- $$$ Dior No-Age Age Defense Refining Crème with SPF 8
- $$$ Sisley Botanical Intensive Day Cream

**Baumann's Choice:** Clinique Superdefense SPF 25 Age Defense Moisturizer

## RECOMMENDED EVENING MOISTURIZERS

- $ Heritage Casto-Vera Cream
- $ Nivea Soft Moisturizing Cream
- $ Aveeno Ageless Vitality Restorative Night Treatment
- $$ Atopalm MLE Cream
- $$ Avon Solutions Maximum Moisture Night Cream
- $$ Biotherm Aquasource Non-Stop Oligo-Thermal Cream Intense Moisturization for Dry Skin
- $$ Clinique Youth Surge Night Age Decelerating Night Moisturizer
- $$ Vivite Replenish Hydrating Cream
- $$ Estée Lauder Hydra Complete Multi-Level Moisture Creme
- $$ Fresh Creme Ancienne Exceptionally Rich Moisturizing Cream
- $$ Osmotics Intensive Moisture Therapy
- $$$ Philosophy Miracle Worker Miraculous Anti-Aging Moisturizer
- $$$ Lancôme Rénergie Microlift R.A.R.E. Intense Targeted Repositioning Lifter
- $$$ Natura Bisse Facial Cleansing Cream + AHA
- $$$ Sisley Global Anti-Age Extra Rich for Dry Skin

**Baumann's Choice:** Atopalm MLE Cream helps repair the skin's barrier without the greasiness.


## Eye Creams

Eye creams are not absolutely necessary, unless you have excessive dryness under your eyes. In most cases, DRNTs can use their regular daytime or nighttime moisturizer. However, many people prefer to use a separate eye cream, so I've listed some choices below.

If you suffer from puffy eyes, place wet chamomile tea bags, caffeinated tea bags, or slices of cucumber over the eyes for ten minutes.


## RECOMMENDED EYE CREAMS

- $ Avon Anew Ultimate Contouring Eye
- $ Neutrogena Clinical Eye Lift Contouring Treatment
- $$ DDF Nourishing Eye Cream
- $$ Dr. Hauschka Eye Contour Day Cream
- $$ Elizabeth Arden Millenium Eye Renewal Crème

$$ Kinerase Ultra Rich Eye Repair
$$ Philosophy Eye Hope Advanced Anti-Aging Eye Cream
$$$ Estée Lauder Time Zone Eyes Ultra-Hydrating Complex
$$$ Fresh Black Tea Age-Delay Eye Cream
$$$ La Mer Eye Balm

**Baumann's Choice:** Dr. Hauschka Eye Contour Day Cream

## Exfoliation

At-home microdermabrasion creams remove the top dead skin layer that makes skin feel rough and causes it to reflect light poorly, giving you a sallow complexion. These products will help reveal a more radiant skin.

### RECOMMENDED MICRODERMABRASION CREAMS

$ Neutrogena Healthy Skin Rejuvenator Anti-Aging Power Treatment Kit
$ Skin Effects by Dr. Jeffrey Dover Cell² Cell Anti-Aging Exfoliating Cleansing Scrub
$$ Clarins Gentle Exfoliating Refiner
$$ Estée Lauder Idealist Micro-D Deep Thermal Refinisher
$$ 100% Pure Red Wine Resveratrol Scrub + Mask
$$$ Dr. Brandt Microdermabrasion in a Jar
$$$ La Mer the Refining Facial
$$$ Clarisonic Mia Skin Cleansing System - Pink
$$$ Kate Somerville ExfoliKate Intensive Exfoliating Treatment

**Baumann's Choice:** Clarisonic Mia Skin Cleansing System - Pink

## SHOPPING FOR PRODUCTS

There are just a few specific ingredients in skin care products that you need to avoid. But there are moisturizing ingredients you should look for that will give you the maximum benefits. Please visit me at www.skintypesolutions .com to tell me your favorite products that contain the following ingredients.

## RECOMMENDED SKIN CARE INGREDIENTS

### *Occlusive ingredients:*

- Beeswax
- Dimethicone
- Grape seed oil
- Jojoba oil
- Lanolin
- Mineral oil
- Paraffin
- Petrolatum
- Propylene glycol
- Soybean oil (contains genistein)
- Squalene

### *Humectants:*

- Alpha hydroxy acids (lactic acid, glycolic acid)
- Glycerin
- Hyaluronic acid (HA)
- Propylene glycol
- Sorbitol
- Sugars (saccharides)
- Urea

### *To improve the skin's barrier:*

- Aloe vera
- Borage seed oil
- Canola oil
- Ceramide
- Cholesterol
- Cocoa butter
- Colloidal oatmeal
- Dexpanthenol (pro-vitamin $B_5$)
- Evening primrose oil
- Fatty acids
- Jojoba oil
- Niacinamide
- Olive oil
- Safflower oil
- Shea butter
- Stearic acid

## SKIN CARE INGREDIENTS TO AVOID

### *Due to drying:*

- Acetone
- Alcohol such as ethanol, denatured alcohol, ethyl alcohol, methanol, benzyl alcohol, isopropyl alcohol, and SD alcohol

## Sun Protection for Your Skin

You rarely have allergies to sunscreen ingredients, so you can use many of the products on the market. Cream formulations are best because they help moisturize the skin. Facial powders with sunscreen are another option if your skin is a bit more on the combination side with an O/D score above 30. However, if your skin is dry, you may not enjoy the drying feel of powder. For everyday use, SPF 15 protection is enough. However, if you expect to be out in the sun for a long period, as when playing golf or at the beach, use SPF 45 or greater. Look for a product with both UVA and UVB protection that contains Parsol (avobenzone).

### RECOMMENDED SUN PROTECTION PRODUCTS

- $ Cetaphil Daily Facial Moisturizer with SPF 15
- $ Minus-Sol Ivory Facial Sun Protection SPF 30
- $ Neutrogena Age Shield + Repair Anti-Aging Sunblock SPF 55
- $ Purpose Dual Treatment Moisture Lotion with SPF 15
- $$ Clarins Radiance-Plus Self Tanning Cream-Gel
- $$ Clinique Superdefense SPF 25 Age Defense Moisturizer Dry Combination
- $$ Kiehl's Vital Sun Protection Lotion SPF 40
- $$ Laura Mercier Mega Moisturizer Cream with SPF 15
- $$ Origins Out Smart Daily SPF 25

**Baumann's Choice:** Cetaphil Daily Facial Moisturizer with SPF 15

### At Risk in Flight

Flying is tough on the skin. First, high levels of UVA come through airplane windows. Second, low humidity levels in the cabin dry skin out, making wrinkles more obvious.

It's important to protect your skin on an airline, especially if you're a DRNT, because you have dryer skin and less skin pigmentation to protect you from sun exposure.

Here's what I recommend: Always apply sunscreen prior to flying. Simplify your makeup by wearing a waterproof mascara and eyeliner, a moisturizing SPF sunscreen, and a hydrating lip gloss.

## Self-Tanning

Many DRNTs have trouble with self-tanners looking spotty, but using an exfoliating scrub before applying the self-tanner to remove dead skin cells will permit a more even tan.

Look for scrubs that contain alpha hydroxy acids, such as lactic acid or glycolic acid, because these help remove the dead skin cells. Read the ingredients on the label to ensure that you avoid exfoliating scrubs that contain petrolatum and mineral oil. These are occlusive moisturizers, which can keep the dihydroxyacetone from working properly. In addition, the tanners I like best contain antioxidants, which produce a more natural tan that looks less orange-yellow.

After applying your self-tanner, do not use a moisturizer for two hours, since it can interfere with the pigmentation process.

### RECOMMENDED SELF-TANNERS

- $ Neutrogena Build a Tan
- $ Jergens Natural Glow Daily For Medium/Tan Skin Tones Moisturizer, 7.5 fl oz
- $ L'Oreal Body Expertise Sublime Bronze Luminous Self-Tanning Lotion Instant Action
- $$ Clarins Self-Tanning Instant Gel
- $$ TanTowel Plus Full Body Self Tanning Towelettes
- $$ St. Tropez Self Tan Bronzing Mousse
- $$ Fake Bake Self Tanning Lotion
- $$ Origins Faux Glow Self-Tanner
- $$$ Dior Bronze Self-Tanner Shimmering Glow Body

**Baumann's Choice:** All self tanners have the ingredient DHA and the same bad smell.

## Your Makeup

Oil-free foundations are not your best bet, since your resistant, dry skin will benefit from oil rather than be harmed by breakouts. So look for cream- or oil-containing foundations.

Because your skin is dry, powders are unnecessary. Powdered blushes and eye shadows may work, but if they feel too dry, try cream-based eye shadows and blushes. Avoid eye shadow setting creams that contain talc, which will make the eyelid skin look drier. Remove eye makeup with mineral, almond, or jojoba oil. Avoid other eye makeup removers, which may dry out your skin.

Shimmery eye shadows are often made of bismuth, mica, and fish scale that can have sharp edges, which may irritate dry skin or increase a dry appearance. If you have noticed this problem, avoid these products.

### RECOMMENDED FOUNDATIONS

$ CoverGirl CG Smoothers All Day Hydrating Make-Up for Normal to Dry Skin
$$ Bobbi Brown Moisture Rich Foundation SPF 15
$$ Chantecaille Real Skin Foundation
$$ DiorSkin Forever Extreme Wear Flawless Makeup SPF 25
$$$ Giorgio Armani Luminous Silk Foundation
$$$ Chanel Vitalumière Satin Smoothing Creme Makeup with SPF 15
$$$ Laura Mercier Moisturizing Foundation

**Baumann's Choice:** Bobbi Brown Moisture Rich Foundation SPF 15 or DiorSkin Forever Extreme Wear Flawless Makeup SPF 25.

### RECOMMENDED BLUSHES

$ Olay Simply Ageless Sculpting Blush
$ Revlon Cream Blush
$$ Bobbi Brown Sheer Color Cheek Tint
$$ Fresh Blush Cream
$$ M·A·C Cream Color Base or Cheek Hue
$$ Nars Cream Blush
$$$ Clinique Touch Blush

**Baumann's Choice:** M·A·C Cream Color Base or Cheek Hue

### RECOMMENDED EYE SHADOWS

$ Boots No7 Stay Perfect Eye Color Cream
$ Revlon Illuminance Creme Shadow
$$ NARS Duo Cream Eyeshadow
$$ Laura Mercier Eye Basics
$$$ Clinique Touch Base for Eyes

**Baumann's Choice:** Revlon Illuminance Creme Shadow

## Consulting a Dermatologist

Although regular checkups to rule out skin cancer are vital for light-skinned DRNTs, there is no other reason to visit a dermatologist.

No procedures are really necessary for DRNTs. However, you might like to have a microdermabrasion procedure, instead of just using a facial scrub or at-home microdermabrasion product.

## MICRODERMABRASION

In the microdermabrasion procedure, the practitioner uses a machine that sprays microcrystals to remove the upper surface layer of the skin. The procedure takes about twenty minutes and costs about $120. Many dermatologists recommend a series of these. DRNTs could have one monthly or before an important occasion to temporarily improve skin texture and increase radiance.

Though not a necessity, this is a luxury for those who can afford it. For the rest of us, facial scrubs are just fine. (I've never had microdermabrasion in my life. I don't have the time to sit there for twenty minutes when I can do the same thing myself in five minutes in the shower.)

## Ongoing Care for Your Skin

You can't overmoisturize. Put tubes of moisturizer in your home, office, and car. Moisturize, moisturize, moisturize. Your skin loves moisture. Protect your skin from the sun, and decrease sun exposure. Use self-tanners if you want color. Get annual checkups to safeguard you from skin cancer.

## RESOURCES

### LOCATING RECOMMENDED PRODUCTS

To find the products recommended in your chapter, I have made it easy for you. You can log on to my website, www.skintypesolutions.com and enter the product that you are looking for into the search field. It will tell you how to find the product. Alternatively, I suggest you go to some of my favorite websites, including www.drugstore.com, www.sephora.com, and www.skinstore. com. All of these sites have a wide variety of products, and you can easily order from them. You can also buy the products at baumannstore.com; all of the proceeds go to charity.

Most $ products can be found at www.cvs.com, www.drugstore.com, or www.walgreens.com, and in many stores such as CVS, Walmart, Walgreens, Kmart, Duane Reade, Target, and Drug Emporium. Avon has an excellent website, www.avon.com, that has ingredient lists for each product.

Most $$ products can be found at www.zitomer.com, www.skinstore.com, www.skincarerx.com, or www.sephora.com, or in Sephora and Beauty 360 stores. Saksfifthavenue.com has many of the $$$ products, as does www.neiman marcus.com. Many department stores carry $$ products, such as Nordstrom, Macy's, and JCPenney. If you come to Miami Beach, be sure to visit Brownes & Co. on Lincoln Road. Their website is www.brownesbeauty.com.

Most $$$ products are found in department stores like Neiman Marcus, Saks Fifth Avenue, and Bergdorf Goodman. These stores often have websites as well.

### LOCATING SUN-PROTECTIVE CLOTHING

A good selection can be found at www.sunprecautions.com, www.coolibar. com, www.shadyladyproducts.com, and www.tackletogo.com.

LOCATING A DOCTOR

I recommend using only board-certified doctors who are very experienced with botulinum toxins, fillers, and peels. As a dermatologist, I feel that dermatologists have the most experience in this area. However, there are many oculoplastic surgeons, facial plastic surgeons, maxillofacial surgeons, and plastic surgeons skilled at these procedures as well. Use the websites below or call these organizations to find reputable doctors in your area. You can find lists of my favorite doctors by city at www.skintypesolutions.com

To find a board-certified dermatologist, contact:
The American Academy of Dermatology: 888-462-DERM and www.aad.org
The American Society for Dermatologic Surgery: 847-956-0900 and www.asds-net.org

To find a dermatologist specializing in skin of color, contact:
The Skin of Color Society: 800-460-9252 and www.skinofcolorsociety.org

To find a cosmetic surgeon, contact:
American Society for Aesthetic Plastic Surgery: 888-272-7711 and www.surgery.org
American Society of Plastic Surgeons: 888-475-2784 and www.plasticsurgery.org
American Academy of Cosmetic Surgery: 312-981-6760 and www.cosmeticsurgery.org
American Academy of Facial Plastic and Reconstructive Surgery: 703-299-9291 and www.aafprs.org

To share your favorite product recommendations with me please log on to www.skintypesolutions.com. At this site you can also find out more information about new skin care products, sign up for updates on what is new, register for online research projects, and share your thoughts on this book. I want to hear how *The Skin Type Solution* helped you! You can follow us at www.facebook.com/BaumannCosmetic or www.Twitter.com/BaumannCosmetic or www.Youtube.com/BaumannCosmetic.

Thanks for your participation in this exciting skin phenomenon!

Leslie Baumann, M.D.

# INDEX

## A

acanthosis nigricans, 280

acne

contributing factors, 16

dryness and, 216

handling breakouts, 76–77

ingredients to use and avoid, 59–60, 80–81, 97, 203–4, 238–39

Intense Pulsed Light (IPL), 242

makeup, 83–84

masks, 236

regimens and products, 55, 72, 74, 76–77, 91–93, 108–11

actinic keratosis, 296

aging, 21, 50, 175–76. *See also specific skin types*

AHAs (alpha hydroxy acids), 270, 299–300, 323

airplane travel, 193, 229, 246–47, 322

alcohol, 275, 284, 290

allergies. *See also* sensitive skin (S)

facial redness, 105

ingredients to avoid, 81, 239

nickel, 105

skin barrier and, 245–46

*vs.* irritant rashes, 204

alpha hydroxy acids (AHA), 270, 299–300, 323

antioxidants

inflammation, 198, 284

ingredients to use, 96–97

toners, 163–64

wrinkles, 128–29, 160, 267, 270, 300–301

ashiness, 193, 208, 281–82, 284, 312–13

Asians, 211–12, 222–23, 280–82. *See also* ethnic or racial background; pigmented skin

atopic dermatitis. *See* eczema

## B

basal cell carcinoma (BCC), 20, 106–7, 175, 296–97

benzoyl peroxide, 75, 77, 97–98, 110–11

blacks, 281–82. *See also* ethnic or racial background; pigmented skin (P)

blushes, 222, 240–41, 257, 324

body moisturizers, 288–89, 303–4

Botox, 24, 63, 102, 124, 137, 160–61, 231

## ABOUT THE AUTHOR

LESLIE BAUMANN, M.D. founded the University of Miami, Division of Cosmetic Dermatology in 1997, which was the first university-run research center dedicated to issues in cosmetic dermatology and skin care. In addition to *The Skin Type Solution,* her book *Cosmetic Dermatology* (McGraw Hill) is the bestselling cosmetic dermatology textbook worldwide and is available in many languages. Her revolutionary skin typing system has been adopted worldwide. Dr. Baumann has forged close working relationships with the world's leading cosmetic and pharmaceutical companies that produce and market products for facial care. She has been on the advisory board or has collaborated on research for more than fifty-two companies. She has written numerous textbook chapters, scientific publications, and newspaper articles on skin care ingredients, in addition to being a regular contributor for Yahoo!Health. Dr. Baumann lives with her husband and children in Miami Beach, Florida.